A
LIFE
with Good Health

John Chun 11/07/22

John Chun

ISBN 978-1-63844-622-4 (paperback)
ISBN 978-1-63844-623-1 (digital)

Christian Faith Publishing, Inc.
832 Park Avenue
Meadville, PA 16335
www.christianfaithpublishing.com

Printed in the United States of America

CONTENTS

PREFACE

This is a book about how to live healthy and long. In other words, this is a book of good health.

The best formula that I can offer you to live healthy and long is following three things, followed by another easy three things. Altogether, there are six things, i.e., elements—which are not many— along with your secrets if you have one or two or more. Out of those six, some are easier than the others, and some are somewhat difficult compared to the others. But none of them is too hard to achieve the goal. Exercise might be a bit hard compared to the rest but could be and would be fun when you begin to see positive results.

Anything is possible, only if you have three Ds: devotion, dedication, and determination for yourself—nothing else. With three Ds, nothing is impossible. Every one of us can do it. So let it be, and let's do it. And we will all be living healthy and long. Why not? We can do it.

If I did it and have been doing it, then certainly you can do it. The first three things are:

1. exercise, the most important of all,
2. drink water wisely, and
3. sleep well.

Then next three are:

4. take one baby aspirin in the morning,
5. take one acid controller (Pepcid) at night, and
6. keep oral hygiene from good to excellent.

So here comes the formula 1 that I created: good health = exercise + water + sleep + baby aspirin + acid controller + oral hygiene.

It is important to stay healthy until the time comes when the One who sent us here finally calls us to come home, a time for us to "fade away" as General MacArthur once said in his farewell speech. Mostly, what I'm dealing with in this book is physical health. And at the end, I'll give you my ideas on how to go back home to where we were before we came into this world. And mental health are the psychiatrist's, psychologist's, or priest's job, not mine. But long time ago, someone said, "Sound mind, sound body," which means physical and mental health go hand in hand.

About forty years ago, I came to America, the land of opportunities, as a young man with no fear. Forty years later, it is time for me to return the favor to America. I devoted all my professional life as an internist treating sick people, many of whom with one ailment or two, sometimes many. Now I'm going to leave that responsibility to the physicians of the next generations, who have more knowledge and better ideas than I do.

Throughout this book, I'm advocating on unhealthy people to become healthy ones and on healthy ones to remain healthy or become healthier. So this book is good news for those who are forty years and older, healthy or not healthy. I do not mind at all young people in their thirties and twenties joining this good news group. Why not? It's good news to all of us! The sooner, the better.

Even though I claimed my book is a book of good news of six, I do admit that some of the readers may find my book boring to read because I do not have any talent in writing books. I'm a scientist, a doctor, not a writer. So for those bored readers of mine, I'm giving you a very important and valuable incentives, i.e., rewards, especially those who want to lose some weight, which is in chapter 12: "How to Lose Weight: The One and Only and the Best." You will not be disappointed and will be well compensated for your precious time and hard-earned money to buy and read this perhaps boring book of mine, I promise.

CHAPTER 1

Health

Certainly, we have to be healthy, regardless of age (young or old) or gender (lady or gentleman). No question about it.

It breaks my heart when I see the tall and huge parking structures of the University of Michigan Hospitals filled up with countless vehicles going up and down, waiting to see if someone leaves. They have to be there because they have a reason or two or more to be there. So let us do something before it is too late. But as we grow older, health becomes more and more and ever more important and moves to the top priority of our lives.

When we were young, being healthy was not so important, something that always remained at the bottom of all the priorities and was one of those things that we took for granted. Those days, we were healthy anyway. Of course, with age, health becomes more important than money or fame. You cannot buy good health with money, and certainly not with fame.

In this book, I'm going to show exactly how we can live healthy and long so that my way becomes your way and then my way and your way become our way. Hopefully, with our way, we all live long and healthy together. That's the goal of this book, which is healthy life.

So far, I have been busy helping people who are physically sick. My goal was and has been totally devoted to treat the disease. Win or lose, life or the other side, it was a struggle with and against diseases.

But from now on, my goal is going to be different. Maybe a lot different. It will be a drastic transformation of some kind. Because now I'm treating people, not the disease.

I'm going to look for you the answer to this important question, "How to live healthy and long?"

Basically, in this book, I'm going to focus on how to be and remain healthy. And then in between those chapters, I'm going to talk about traveling and a few social issues with which you and I can have differences of opinion. For that, let's get ready to agree to disagree.

When we are talking about healthy living, many people immediately consider something like magic water or mysterious pill or strange food, etc. In reality, many people invest and waste lots of money and precious time just doing exactly what I said above, looking for magic rather than a true solution.

In that regard, we can immediately think of someone whose name is Emperor Qin Shi Huang of ancient China, who became famous for the pursuit of eternal youth through medicinal herbs, i.e., some sort of magic. He sent out his generals and soldiers throughout the country and abroad, looking for the magic. And when they came back to him empty-handed, no one survived the emperor's fury, and so no one came out of the emperor's palace alive. Through him, we learned valuable lessons, that such an effort has its own limit, which is failure and waste of time and money at the end.

Unfortunately, recent study showed that our aging process begins at the age of twenty-six. In other words, ever since we were born into this world, we are marching toward youth. And then at the age of twenty-six, we all stop becoming any younger. Instead, we are all marching toward the opposite direction of what we have been doing, i.e., aging. We put our first steps toward aging, i.e., degenerative changes, at such a young age of only twenty-six, and then we will not get any younger until we die.

As we all know, these degenerative changes—i.e., aging—is very much insidious that the process is so slow and almost unrecognizable, sometimes invisible. On top of it, it's our human nature to deny anything we do not like. It is this mental defense mechanism of denial that makes it very difficult for us to see the truth. But at the moment, we recognize it with our own eyes. Let's be sensitive and truthful and do something about it, instead of hiding behind denial, cosmetics, Botox, and cosmetic surgery, etc.

We may not recognize aging until the age of forties or fifties if we are lucky with the magical help of denial and makeups. But the truth will remain with us forever. It shows itself slowly but surely when the time comes, no matter how strongly we may refuse to accept. You can deny anything or everything. But you cannot deny the truth. The truth always prevails at the end.

Before it's too late, I have to mention briefly and clearly that there are two different kinds of truths in our world—the truth that will never change no matter what and the truth that changes with time. Even though we do not want to change what we believe, sometimes we have no choice but to.

The best example of the first is that the sun rises from the east and goes down to the west. The best example of the second is that the world used to be flat. But not anymore. Not now. It used to be flat not too long ago. But it is round now. If someone claims the earth is flat, even kindergarten children will laugh and laugh until their faces turn blue, a sign of hypoxia. But it used to be flat, until one scientist in Italy was put to jail or on house arrest simply because he announced the earth is round, not flat. The one who told the truth suffered the consequences of telling the truth that is not the truth any longer. What an irony!

But even in the twenty-first century of the modern world, there are societies where humans are not treated equally. There are some people, although small in number, who believe we humans are born different and should be treated differently. You must have heard and known about racism, sexism, and so on. We in America came a long way in this regard, but we still have to go a long way ahead. Please, America, let's move forward, not backward. Our time is too precious to waste. Going backward is unacceptable. Whether you like it or not, when the truth changes, we have no choice but to change accordingly.

But many people have a problem with this second example of truth. Just remember, when someone was telling the truth about the shape of the earth, the entire society with the help of the church went after him, took him to the court, and put him on house arrest.

Even in the Bible, which is filled with the truth, we have to have the wisdom and honesty and flexibility to recognize that there are two kinds of truth—one that will never change and the other that already changed or that will change or has to change with time in the future. Sometimes even though something written in the Bible changed or has to change, many of us do not have the wisdom to change ourselves or accept the truth that needs to change. And consider the fact that the Bible was written more than two thousand years ago by people just like you and me who make mistakes right and left. We all know that the gospels of the Bible were not written by Jesus himself and not even by his disciples. It was written by the second or third generations of disciples. The gospels were written by people who'd never seen Jesus but only heard of him from someone else.

Always remember that the Bible is not perfect either if we consider who wrote it and when it was written. Being written by the people, i.e., disciples of the disciples, especially in the New Testament, who had a lot less education than us—many of whom received no formal education at all—and who did not have computer, iPad, or iPhone. Almost all the disciples of Jesus, and even Jesus himself, are deadly poor, uneducated, outside of the mainstream of their own society, etc., compared to other religious leaders, such as Muhammad or Buddha. As you know and as we all know, the Bible was not written by Jesus who created his religion called Christianity neither by his disciples, compared to other religions. It was written by someone without any firsthand knowledge of the Creator. How do we believe a book—the way it is written by people who are second or third generations of the disciples—is only the truth, nothing but the truth?

If you insist that the Bible was written by the Holy Spirit and say we have no choice but to accept and believe the way it's written, then we have a problem. You and I have a so-called difference of opinion. Yes, we have a problem. But do you remember we agreed to disagree?

There is another reason why it is dangerous to believe or teach the Bible the way it is written without digesting. Simply, think when we eat the foods, what happens if we swallow or dump the foods into the stomach without chewing? What will happen to our stomach and ultimately to our body and our health? What will happen if we put the teachings of Jesus directly? For example, in the very famous teaching in the Gospel of John where Jesus said to his disciples, "I am the way, and the truth, and the life; no one comes to the Father but through me. Oneness with Father," does this mean that only Christians will see the Father in heaven? Then what happens to those people who did not know him in the past or who do not know him at the present day? What happens to people of other religions? The answer will come out in the final chapter "Conclusion" briefly.

Going back to the main issue of health, aging—i.e., degenerative changes—unfortunately seems to belong to the first group of the truth. I sincerely hope this one becomes or moves to the second group in the future. But it is simply a hope that does not seem to change. So there seems to be no hope as far as I know. We cannot change or reverse aging. On the surface, the skin gets wrinkles all over, starting from our beautiful and handsome face. The height itself shrinks. On top of it, the spine bends forward, a sign of humility perhaps. And your beautiful hair turns gray or disappears slowly like mine. And so on.

It is quite unfair to have changes externally, but there will be universal changes—meaning, we age inside as well, which means wherever blood vessels go, our body will undergo degenerative changes. There is no exception inside or out. When we age, we all age everywhere physically and mentally, visibly and invisibly.

When we become old, such an illness like common cold or flu or even simple fatigue, etc., which never bothered us before when we were young, will make certain to make our lives miserable and make their presence known. On top of that, accumulated stresses throughout our difficult life, in combination with degenerative changes, make our lives even more difficult. It used to be none of my concern in the past when I was young. It used to be someone else's problem, not mine, when I was growing up. But now it is my problem too.

Anyway, modern science or advanced modern medicine is absolutely unable to give us any solution to reverse the natural course of degenerative changes, i.e., aging. At least, in our generation or in the next ten generations or so, there will be no solution for this delicate and mysterious problem. Not even we can see the solution on the horizon in the twenty-first century. Probably, no matter how advanced our science might be, this will remain forever unsolved as the mystery of the human body. We would be better off if there is no solution for this. This is the reason why.

Let's suppose somebody, a crazy scientist, found the solution for the aging process. Then what happens if all the people of the world know the secret and remain young? If only a few of us own the fountain of youth, it seems there will be no problem. But just imagine how the world would look like if everybody knows the big secret of eternal youth.

As a matter of fact, like the movie produced by Steve Spielberg, *Back to the Future*, if we can freely go to the future and the past and come back and forth with a vehicle that looks like an automobile, what will happen? What kind of world will we be living? Suddenly, if our ancestors of the civil war era show up in front of us with a lot-younger-looking men or women than me or my children, what kind of family issues do we have to deal with? My grandfather looks a lot younger than I do. And the other way around. What if I myself show up in front of my great-great-great-grandchildren with much younger looks than them, who will be the old or young generation of this "dysfunctional" family? Who will be in charge of my perhaps "reversed" or "upside-down" family? Who is senior? Who is junior? How do we call one another? How do I call my father, whose physical age is much younger and who is intellectually much immature than I am, or my son, who is older and much more mature than his grandfather? What is going on here?

Another way to solve the problem of aging is like what happens in the movie *The Curious Case of Benjamin Button* starring Brad Pitt, whose character became an ugly old man in the middle of the movie and then suddenly one day reversed the course of aging by gradually becoming younger and younger and finally becoming a newborn baby at the end of the movie. So the best solution for this question, in my opinion, instead of looking for the cure, would be that we have to turn this unavoidable and undesirable bad friend—i.e., aging process—into a manageable living partner of our lives and move forward.

As we are intellectually becoming old and wise, we all learn to accept this reality the way it is and move on. Getting old has to be a learning process to achieve the ultimate maturity and wisdom of our lives, making a choice between "just fade away" and "just die" at the end.

As a matter of fact, aging—i.e., degenerative changes—or ultimately the issue of death does not have to be our worst enemy or unavoidable curse imposed by the Creator of the universe. Rather, we have to turn what appears to be the curse of an angry God into a blessing of a loving God.

In that sense, General Douglas MacArthur's farewell speech to America makes so much sense to all of us, or at least to me, which is "Old soldiers never die; they just fade away." Yes, we are. Let's not die, as in "to be or not to be" by Shakespeare. We all are soldiers of a tough life, who will just fade away at the end. We are not going to die at the end. Rather, we just fade away. When the curtain comes down from above with the stage getting darker slowly, we just fade away quietly without making any noise.

Simply because we were not the ones who made the decision to come into this world, that does not mean that we have to die without any consideration of our own decision or feeling. But at the end, we do have the choice to just fade away on our own way. That's how we die. We may not be able to control "when," but we can definitely do something about "how" we just die or just fade away. My question is not "to be or not to be," like someone who lived and said in England long time ago, who happens to be a much better writer than I am. Actually, the question is "Are we going to die or just fade away?" That is my question. That's got to be your question too. But I know which one you choose. Certainly, I know which one I choose.

We always have to imagine what kind of shape we are in physically and mentally when we fade away. Hopefully, I can and will give you the answer on the physical aspect. For the other part, you need to seek help from psychiatrists, ministers, priests, Buddhist monks, or psychologists. One of the books that you should look into would be the Bible. But always remember, "Sound mind, sound body."

I'll try to give you my answer throughout this book. Or let's find the answer together.

We are not a mere presence here on earth and then disappear helplessly and hopelessly at the end. We all have to choose how to just fade away when the time comes. When the stage of our lives gradually darkens and the curtain comes down slowly from above, accepting that our time finally has arrived, then we just fade away to meet the One who sent us into this wonderful world.

Are we going to fade away happily or sadly or with regret or with hope? The choice is yours and mine. We may have no control over "when." But definitely and positively, we can choose "how." Yes, absolutely and positively, we can do something about "how."

So aging itself—furthermore, the issues of death—is not the tyranny of a revenging, angry, and/or punishing God. It is our efforts that we are in the process of connecting the dots in our lives, and it is a part of our learning process of finding everlasting love and blessings of the living and loving God.

We need to have the wisdom to turn this aging process, i.e., the bad friend, into our good partner of life, i.e., blessing as we grow older and older until the time finally comes. So don't waste your hard-earned money and precious time given by God chasing after proven lies. Come along with me to see if we can find a truth or two together so that we maintain our good health as we grow older.

Here, I'm going to introduce to you the six elements—factors, however I call—that will show us how to digest the degenerative changes, i.e., aging, on our behalf and live long and healthy until the time that we just fade away.

1. Exercise appropriately for your body.
2. Drink water wisely.
3. Sleep well.

I recommend three more, as all those are very easy to do. Every one of you must follow these two sets of advice, along with others.

4. Take one baby aspirin in the morning.
5. Take one Pepcid in the evening.
6. And the last but not the least, keep the inside of your mouth clean.

In short, the formula of good health that I invented looks like this: good health = exercise + water + sleep + baby aspirin + acid controller + oral hygiene.

Although it is not my area of expertise, I had to include dental hygiene because it's so important. You know I'm not a dentist, but I'll do my best to prove my point and give you the solution.

On each chapter of health-related issues, including "How to Lose Weight: The One and Only and the Best," except "Water," I always made sure to put the solution at the end. Some answers come a bit sooner in each chapter, but I always put the solutions toward the end of each chapter. Without the solutions, my book is useless.

When I talk about exercise, I'm going to discuss why we have to exercise, which exercise is good or better than the other that will give us the best result to our body, and how to achieve the goal. I'm going to give you the "why," "which," and "how."

When I talk about water, I'm going to discuss what kind of water is good for our body and how we can make good water to the best one for our body.

When I talk about sleep, I'm going to discuss what is the best way to have good sleep and about sleep disorder in general and how to treat the problem of insomnia, one of the worst enemies of our good health.

When I talk about aspirin and Pepcid, I'm going to discuss the reason why we have to take these two.

When I talk about dental hygiene, I'm going to discuss extensively how we can and what is the better or best way to eliminate gum disease, along with halitosis, i.e., bad breath.

At the end of each chapter of the above six, I always make sure to mention how to solve the problem in the most effective way. If I do not give the answer, dump this book where it belongs, the trash can.

On top of the six elements, I also included the chapter "How to Lose Weight: The One and Only and the Best." And for all those who want to lose weight, this chapter will be another good news, hopefully, one of the best news you will ever encounter.

I hope my solution is the best and the one and only for all of us.

CHAPTER 2

Travel

Being second to the last of eight siblings, that's who I was and still am. I have three older brothers and three older sisters but only one younger brother, who is six years younger than I am. I'm so lucky to have him as my younger brother.

Having too many bosses, I always wanted peace and quiet alone and away from the noises and bosses. In order to find a getaway solution for peace and quiet on my own, I chose traveling all by myself or with a few of my best friends.

I had too many bosses in my early life. But don't misunderstand. I love my parents, my brothers, and my sisters. As I grow older and older, I miss my mom and daddy more than ever. I love all my four brothers and three sisters. Particularly and most of all, I love my younger brother, who became the youngest for me.

But I had to find my own freedom in the middle of nowhere, such as at the top of a mountain or on the quiet but sometimes noisy sand dunes next to the angry ocean. You know that Korea is a peninsula, surrounded by an ocean, except the northern part, with 70 percent mountains. I loved the space that a small tent provides for only one person or two, three at most. I fell in love with the feeling of liberty and freedom the moment I step out of my house.

But the farther I get away from home, the closer and more appreciative I feel about everything I have—my home, my parents, my friends, etc. Even though I am far away from home, I feel ever

17

closer to everything that I have. So by the time I return home after each travel, I become a better person to my family and friends and ultimately to the community where I belong. Probably, that might be the reason why I fell in love with traveling deeper and deeper.

When I was growing up, it was a "boys never cry" culture. Under any circumstances, no matter how I feel, I should not show my perhaps "precious" tears in front of anyone. But lately, there were several occasions while traveling that I became a little bit emotional so that I came close to showing tears in my eyes—once in Egypt, Rome, and Alaska. I cannot explain why. It is impossible for me to put it in writing. By now, you all know I'm not a good writer. So the best way I can suggest or describe is that you, every one of you, visit the same places I went and hopefully feel the same at least or deeper than I did.

When we travel, we will have two different feelings about those places we visited during and at the end of the journey. The first is a place that you want to go back to again and again as many times as possible. In those places, you feel like you will find something new to enlighten your soul and that never fails to give something. In my mind, I have four places like that: Rome, Egypt, Alaska, and Barcelona. The second is a place that is good to visit but not good enough to make you want to come back again and again. Unfortunately, those places in my list are any places other than the above four.

I'd like to travel alone or only with a few. There is an advantage and a disadvantage on both traveling alone or with a few and in a group. It all depends on how you take the most of the advantage out of both, by doing research and studying the place where you are going. For example, you will learn a lot more about the history, people, and culture in such places like Rome and Alaska if you travel alone or with a few. And yet in such places like Egypt, it would be better traveling in a group with a travel guide. But it all depends on your personality and inclination.

Like anything else in our lives, you have to be healthy first to be able to travel a lot. That is the bottom line, unfortunately. In the meantime, work hard and save enough money. And when you have time to travel, take off and go wherever you want to go, starting with the place where you want to go the most.

You cannot imagine how happy you are when you are planning and thinking about the travel whichever way that you know the best. Just thinking about it makes me happy and excited.

Sometimes when you are traveling, not only you will see places you have never seen before and meet people you have never met before, but when and if you are lucky enough, you will taste a food you have never tasted before, even though you can eat all kinds of ethnic foods of many different cultures inside America. You, especially your tongue, will remember a long, long time the taste of some of the food you experienced while traveling. I'm going to give you the lists that are printed in my memory, especially in my tongue as well.

Roasted chicken of Lisbon, Portugal

The whole chicken just got out of propane gas grill. I do not know how it was marinated. But once I started putting it into my mouth, I felt like I was in heaven.

I like turkey but never liked chicken in my entire life. I've seen some people who do not like chicken on the table for the same reason just like me.

I grew up in a city or town where a big marketplace was located nearby my house. When I was growing up, I had seen so many chickens being butchered with no mercy at all. So many times, I saw them dying and bleeding when I was passing by to go to school. I could not eat cooked chicken on the table at home or anywhere else. I did not know the reason why until I grew up to be in the late twenties or early thirties of my life. I have a mild case of posttraumatic stress disorder (PTSD). But the funny thing is, even after I found out the reason, my problem with chicken continued or even got worse sometimes. I can safely say it got better when I faced the reality and tried to understand my problem. I was able to stop the bleeding, and the wound got better, but the scar remains. Is it too much to ask that the scar goes away also? The bleeding stopped, and the wound healed, but the scar remains. I still feel sorry for those chickens who died to please us, including myself. I like to eat turkey than chicken because I have never seen any turkey being butchered by humans, one of us. So I cannot enjoy chicken because I had PTSD, and I am still going through childhood trauma. I know it is not bleeding anymore, but I still have the scar. I seldom eat chicken but only the fried one, such as Kentucky Fried Chicken or Popeyes, only the extra crispy one.

This one in Lisbon broke my heart that chickens are tasting this good, even to my tongue. But it was the best chicken I have ever eaten in my entire life.

Tofu *zigae* of Anchorage, Alaska

The soup (*zigae*) is made with soft tofu, mixed with seafood and then boiled in a very hot temperature on top of a propane gas flame. You can request it to be done mild, moderate, or very hot—I mean spicy hot. Of course, I always ask very hot. As you expect, I eat this Korean dish many, many times, and I like it a lot. Among all this dish from Korean restaurants in America, and Korea included, this was the best.

There is one Korean restaurant in Los Angeles specializing in this particular dish, which I had visited on several occasions. It is really good. But the one in Anchorage is number 1, the best on my list. And I want to emphasize that taste is subjective, not objective. I hope the chef or the owner in Los Angeles understands and accepts the second place because his *zigae* is a very close second.

Barbecued ribs of Yellow Stone National Park

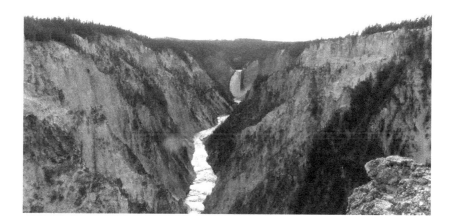

There is a small town just outside the north gate of Yellow Stone National Park. I do not remember the name of the town. I forgot the name of the restaurant too.

At the end of the day, we were looking for a place to have a nice dinner. We were hungry. You know better than I do about what is barbecued ribs and how it is cooked. So there is no need to explain what it is. We found a restaurant with a small line outside, which means it's good. We immediately knew it's a good one. People who were leaving looked so happy with a big smile. It did not take us long to find out how good the food was. Their specialty was barbecued ribs. We all agreed to come back the next day, which we did. It was the best on my list, which is very short. Every one of us said that it was our best.

Seafood taco

It happened while in San Juan, Puerto Rico. It just happened out of nowhere. We were walking around the street and got hungry. Time to have lunch. We all did not expect that we were going to meet the best, not one of the best. We found a decent restaurant on a busy street and ordered seafood taco with no expectation whatsoever. We only followed the waitress's advice. Then the unexpected happened out of nowhere.

To be honest, I ate taco a lot, but no seafood taco before, always ground beef taco. Actually, I had no seafood taco in my entire life. It was for the first time and my last so far. I could not find any better one. And it was the best and is still the best so far.

It's water, not food

In Canadian Rocky, there is one place you have a chance to go near the glacier. Actually, you can go on the top of it with the special vehicle you see on the Discovery Channel and walk around on the top of the glacier. There is a small creek, and you can drink the water from it, which I cannot describe how good the taste is.

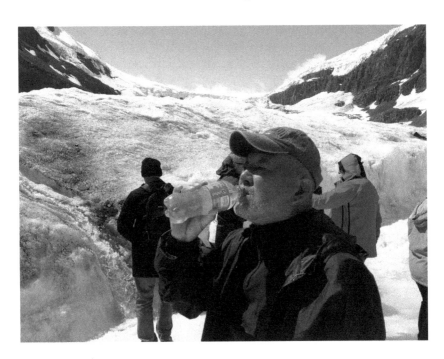

Of course, water does not have any particular taste. It is the feeling. It was so good that I did not want to leave the glacier, but my time was too short. I came down with a bottle of glacier water in my car.

A few hours later, I drank the same water, but the feeling was different. You have to drink the glacier water on the top of the glacier with the same temperature from the creek to have the same feeling that I had on the top of the glacier. That's why you need to go and travel the world your way or my way. No one can do it for you.

I'll talk more about this water and other water in the chapter "Water."

Although it makes me very happy just to talk about it, please remember that I'm not an expert in traveling, not even close, and not to mention my writing skill as well.

CHAPTER 3

Exercise,
the Most Important of All

Although there are so many different and good exercises around us in this world, we have to find the most proper exercise for ourselves. As a matter of fact, one of the main goals of writing this book is to help you readers find the best exercise that is available and most easily accessible to you while costing minimally. Then what kind of changes will the exercise bring to us other than muscle mass increase?

The exercise that I'm about to talk about is not the kind that only professional athletes are able to do or are doing. It is about the kind of exercise for anyone and that everyone can do unless the person is handicapped by either a congenital condition (born with) or acquired condition (happened after birth) that keep them from doing it. Then we have to come up with a certain exercise which is proper and appropriate for that particular individual.

Even though you are someone who is handicapped from birth or after birth, it does not matter. You have to find an exercise that fits you. Even a person in a wheelchair can play basketball. Nothing is impossible. Likewise, it has to be something that we all can do one way or another.

Even though we do the same kind of exercise, we can have different results. Even though we do the same kind of exercise, depending on the physical condition of the person, it can be exercise or the opposite, which is waste of time and money.

Sometimes, even if we use the same group of muscles, the result would be different other than exercise, i.e., called labor. For a one-year-old baby, walking itself would be a vigorous exercise, but for a grown-up healthy adult, it is not enough exercise at all. After one hour of walking outside in the neighborhood, if a healthy young adult claims that he had a good exercise, there is a serious problem. For a young person with a heart condition or chronic lung disease, walking itself could be a good and vigorous exercise. But for a healthy young person, it cannot be a good exercise but may be a stress reliever with a bunch of fresh air at best. For an elderly person, walking itself could be a good exercise. But for the young and healthy, they will achieve a desired result with vigorous exercise, which is much more vigorous than walking.

Then what is true exercise? The answer comes next.

Respiratory Alkalosis

The true face of exercise should be that all the muscles involved are pushed to the limit of their ability, then begging to the owner, who is soaked in a profuse sweating, "Please I cannot go on any longer. I cannot breathe. Please stop." Sweating all over the face and body is the way true exercise looks like and should be.

So when we work out, we have to have shortness of breath, sweat a lot, and last at least more than thirty minutes, hopefully an hour or so. And you need a short break, i.e., rest, in between.

If the workout is too easy, the effort will be wasted. If it is too vigorous, the chance of getting injury will be high. Always stay within your limit; never go over your limit. Only you know your limit, no one else.

This is my definition of exercise. True workout should be for my own health. In the process of exercise, all the muscles involved are exhausted, so our muscles have to demand much more oxygen than usual to meet the physiological demand of oxygen in muscles.

Our two lungs have to function to the maximal limit. As a result, our lungs bring the maximal amount of oxygen into the bloodstream, then into the cells of our body. At the same time, the carbon dioxide—i.e., the end product of an extremely increased metabolism due to exercise—will be pushed out through the lungs. As result of this high-powered exchange of the two gases—uptake of oxygen and expulsion of carbon dioxide in the lungs—our body will undergo a metabolic transformation from an acidic environment (acidosis) to an alkalotic environment (alkalosis). Scientifically speaking, we call this phenomenon respiratory alkalosis because alkalosis in this particular environment is caused by respiration by the lungs. In other words, with true exercise, through vigorous respiration, our entire body transforms into an alkalotic state from an acidotic state. Respiratory alkalosis is the goal of true exercise.

Wait! There is another one.

Endorphin

There is another important element related with true exercise, i.e., true workout.

While we are dipping into true exercise, sometimes we get into a strange experience or a feeling like "What is going on?" or "What is happening today?" Finally, you ask yourself, "Why is it so easy today?" Exercise seems so easy. It has to be hard, but one should not feel tired or have shortness of breath. As professional athletes often describe, they go into a so-called groove. It is hard to describe the feeling. Perhaps feeling high. Have you heard about the so-called runner's high? Everything becomes easy. We would not feel tired at all during or after a strenuous workout. We don't have to breathe fast, and there are no shortness of breath and no muscle ache. As a matter of fact, our breathing slows down, your heart rate as well. Our mind becomes calm, rather than excited.

The moment when we experience this kind of "high" feeling is when our body produces a mysterious substance called endorphin.

The pituitary gland, which is located deep inside our brain, is the one producing endorphin. That's why we feel high.

Actually, we—everyone like you and me or any average, ordinary person—can produce this substance. That precious substance does not belong to professional athletes only. We all can produce the substance. When and if we are going through true exercise, we all produce it, at the same time when our body transforms from acidosis to alkalosis. Most likely, the alkalosis triggers the production of endorphin. This is the goal of exercise—to make our body become alkalotic and produce endorphin subsequently. Research showed it has a similar molecular structure, so it was named similarly. To emphasize it is produced inside our body, scientists put "endo" in front of the name and "orphin" at the end, as in morphine, which become endorphin. This morphinelike substance does not cost any money but only requires true exercise.

When we start producing endorphin from our pituitary gland, like a person who received a small dose of morphine from outside, similar phenomena will occur in our body. Our heart rate goes down; our blood pressure goes down, and breathing goes down. We become very calm and cozy. We do not feel much pain when injured during a strenuous exercise due to the analgesic effect of morphine. Oh no, not morphine but analgesic effect of endorphin.

The person feels that he moves slowly. But in reality, he is moving very fast and can move as fast as he can or even faster than ever. The person even does not feel that much shortness of breath as he should. His heart does not beat as fast as it should; his heart doesn't have to and even beats slowly, i.e., bradycardia. As a result, he doesn't get exhausted. Instead, his opponent gets tired out and burns out. Look at Michael Jordan. He is the best example of endorphin at work. His story comes next.

So I make formula 2: true exercise = respiratory alkalosis + endorphin. This is the goal of exercise, true workout.

Pistons, Bulls, and Michael Jordan

There are few superheroes in professional sports in our generation. Actually, more than few. But for sure, Michael Jordan (MJ) is one of them. He is the living example of endorphin at work. When we look at him running up and down the basketball court, we are witnessing endorphin itself. You see him sweating, but you never see him out of breath.

Stars of stars are playing against one another at the NBA Finals, tied with three games each in the final seventh game, with a few seconds remaining in the fourth quarter, and with his team two points behind. And with his teammate inbounding the ball, he picked up the ball. As soon as he shot and the ball left his hands, the game clock expired. You know the rest of the story.

The best defensive player of the opposing team was defending him closely one on one. In addition, the players on the right and left—three out of the five players of the opposing team—were all over him. And everybody in the stadium—literally everybody, including people rooting for the home team and the visiting team, players on both side of the bench, etc.—all stood up jumping up and down and screaming at top of their voices. The one and only MJ, under the influence of endorphin, calmly dropped a three-point field goal and sent everybody home in regulation time, no overtime, shaking everybody's head.

He is the one who always comes to the stadium first and leaves the stadium last. His practice starts before the game with the other players but continues after the games also. When the other players are busy in the locker room preparing to go home, he remains at the court and continues his routine.

Thus, the Chicago Bulls of MJ won the NBA champion titles for six times total—three times in row, then one year off, and another three times in a row. He took one year off in the middle because he wanted to be professional baseball player. He tried and failed. What a loser! I'm sorry. I mean as a baseball player. Then he came back. And you know the rest of the story, which will be explained in the chapter "Rome."

Just a little more about professional basketball. To be precise, it is about the Detroit Pistons. Before the heyday of the Chicago Bulls of MJ, the Detroit Pistons had its own peak, a kind of "short" one—two years in a row of NBA championship after losing the NBA Finals to the LA Lakers of Magic Johnson, who is the best professional basketball player of all time in my opinion. Yes, Magic is the best, in terms of athletic ability as he can play all the positions of basketball—guard, forward, and center whenever necessary. But compared to the two of them in terms of achievement, Michael is better. Of course, no one knows if Magic did not retire prematurely. We all know why he had to retire early.

During those two years of the Pistons' peak days, the Bulls of MJ was no match against the Pistons, not even close. Even if he scored more than fifty points, his team still lost to the Pistons. Probably, with those three years of losing badly against the Pistons, MJ must have learned how to lose, and consequently, he had mastered how to win. This is the reason why the Pistons had such an excellent three years of beating up the Bulls and the rest of the NBA teams.

First, the Pistons had Isiah Thomas, the best shooting guard you will ever see, and Joe Dumars, the most excellent defensive guard, who became the president of the Pistons' organization as soon as he retired as a player and who started in one organization and finished his entire career at the same team, which tells what kind of a person he is, not to mention as a player. Isiah Thomas did the same too as a player. Also, here comes Vinnie Johnson, whose nickname was the "Microwave" because he was always ready to score a bunch of points immediately when he comes in the game.

Second, then centers, like Bill Laimbeer. Of course, not only he is tall because he plays center, also he is big. Yes, he is huge so that once he takes his position under the basket, no one can push him around. His father was an investment banker, who is the only father who had more money than his son who is a current professional basketball player. There is another center, Rick Mahorn. He is as huge as Bill Laimbeer or maybe bigger. If another player fouls him, another player will fall on the floor. If he fouls another player, the other player will get hurt. Because of these two players, the Pistons were called "Bad Boys."

Third, all of a sudden and out of nowhere, here came Dennis Rodman. Where did he come from? He started playing regular basketball while in college. His official record tells that the story is true, especially the rate of free throw. Fans were even giving him a standing ovation if he made a free throw. Because he rarely made free throws. But his rebound, both defensive and offensive, is outstanding. No player can match him. He jumps higher than anybody else. He jumps so high that opposing centers lose the battle for the rebound. And he runs faster than anyone else in the court. Have you seen a deer running in the forest?

So MJ and the Bulls are no match for the Pistons at its peak. Joe Dumars covered MJ one on one. Then Dennis Rodman gave a hand. Then the Bulls was no match for the Pistons, like any other NBA teams. But all of a sudden, Rodman moved to Chicago, and you know the rest of the story.

By the way, a few weeks ago, on a TV interview, a former Pistons' teammates said the Pistons was not the same team after Rick Mahorn was transferred to an expansion team from Minnesota. They said the Pistons was like an old tiger with no teeth. No teams were afraid of the Pistons as they were in the past anymore.

Adrenalin

Many people confuse exercise and labor.

Just because you move the same group of muscles and you believe it brings the same kind of results, then it will be a big misunderstanding. Of course, to some extent, exercise can be a labor, and vice versa. Under certain circumstances, such as to bring foods to the table or to make more money out of greed, if it is not for your own health and well-being, it is extremely difficult or almost impossible to initiate to bring respiratory alkalosis along with endorphin.

For example, for some kind of physical activities that a construction worker has to go through day after day, it is highly unlikely that his physical activities will give his body respiratory alkalosis, and subsequently endorphin. His body almost certainly will produce exactly the opposite substance called adrenalin. In these circumstances, it would be a better description to say "labor" rather than "exercise."

As you can imagine, there would be an entirely opposite reaction to our body when our body produces adrenalin from the adrenal glands located on the top of each of our kidney, compared to endorphin from the pituitary gland deep inside our brain.

When adrenalin is circulating in our body, our blood pressure goes up, our heart beats faster, our breathing unnecessarily goes faster, and our mind becomes anxious instead of calm. Of course, there would be a difference between a person who remains in the cubicle all day long while struggling with his computer and a person who works all day outside while lifting heavy machinery. Although there is a significant difference in the amount of muscle activity between these two persons, the motivation and outcome would be entirely different compared to a person who exercises for their own health. So when a construction worker goes to work in the morning, he says to his wife, "I'm going to work," and never say, "I'm going to exercise." Because the mindset of going out to work for money is entirely different from going out for true exercise.

Another example is someone who goes out for golfing and arrives at the golf course just a few minutes before the tee time. Upon arrival, without having time to loosen up the muscles, at the first tee, he hits the ball in a hurry. Then instead of walking, he comfortably rides a powered cart either by gasoline or electric, looks for his ball, parks his cart right behind his ball, then hits the ball again, repeats these activities, and finishes eighteen holes. And then he says to himself, "I had a good workout today." Everybody can see a problem here. A big problem. After wasting his time and money, if the person says, "I did a good exercise," what good did he do to himself? It makes more sense if he felt that a lot of stress got released. In here, do we notice that there is no respiratory alkalosis involved? And no endorphin for sure.

Here is another worse example. To achieve a good exercise and stress release, someone goes to the golf course but comes home not only without true exercise but also with more stress than before. On the green grasses of the field, with cool fresh air and under crystal clear blue sky, we see some people put more stress on themselves with an angry face while betting for money or arguing whether someone violated the Professional Golfers' Association golf rules or cheated or not. We also see someone chain-smoking in between the golf shots. Did I say someone smoking while golfing? What a tragedy!

Once in a while, we hear a sad news that a dedicated amateur golfer, such as you or me, ends up having a sudden heart attack while aiming a crucial short but scary put and die before witnessing his ball goes into the hole. Definitely, I'm not emphasizing that golf itself is bad. It could be an excellent true exercise depending on how you play.

Again, through true exercise, if we move or transform our body from acidosis toward alkalosis, the metabolic syndromes of modern era—such as hypertension, type 2 diabetes, high-LDL cholesterol or bad cholesterol, low-HDL cholesterol or good cholesterol, and abdominal obesity, even coronary artery disease, heart attack, stroke, etc.—that we might want to avoid at all costs will move away and disappear from us because they cannot survive the alkalotic environment of our body along with endorphin produced by true exercise. And we will be able to live as long and healthy as we want. Even cancer will say goodbye and leave us.

Just recently, world-famous oncologists, also known as specialists for cancers, agreed and announced that cancer cells prefer an acidic environment rather than an alkalotic environment. In other words, cancer likes and loves acidosis. Cancer hates alkalosis. In acidosis, cancer thrives in our body. In alkalosis, cancer cannot survive in our body. It leaves our body or dies or disappears.

We have to eliminate the metabolic syndromes listed above as a result of enormous stress and acidosis that we created, which invade our body and are being unrecognized by you and me.

But through good exercise, we give frequent and numerous chances to our body to become an alkalotic environment along with endorphin. As a result, we give our body good strength to fight off and eliminate all those metabolic syndromes as well as cancer. That is the goal of this book, my book.

Last, there is a medical condition other than the metabolic syndromes and cancer that like acidosis and is worse than the metabolic syndromes and cancer. This is the worst of all. This is "death."

We all go through acidosis, which is a natural and inevitable phenomenon that occurs to everybody just before death. In other words, when we die or are about to die, we all go through a condition called metabolic acidosis, along with respiratory acidosis. Both are acidosis. We all die with acidosis. That's the end of all living creatures, human and animal included.

Next, the good news. I'm going to introduce to you the best true exercise among myriads of them, in my opinion. The better news is it does not cost you much, just a little to almost none. As you understand by now, there are three different exercises we can think of.

First, true exercise that produces respiratory alkalosis and endorphin. I explained this already.

Second, semitrue exercise that does not produce the above two extremely crucial elements, which you know very well by now. It might look like exercise externally, but not at all internally. But it is exercise. It produces a bit of alkalosis, but no endorphin in this case. This is where I and most of us belong. We need to put a bit more effort to move up to the first group.

And third, false exercise that produces adrenalin instead of the two—alkalosis and endorphin. It appears to be exercise. Externally, it disguises to be some kind of exercise, but if you look inside it, you are not going to see what you want to see. Instead, you will find something hazardous to our body, which will make our blood pressure, heart rate, blood sugar, and cholesterol go up and will increase our chance to develop coronary artery disease. So I would say it's the opposite of true exercise, which we must avoid at all costs. Fortunately, we, the majority of us, do not belong to the third group, except for a few of us. It externally appears to be an exercise but internally produces the opposite hormone, adrenalin.

True Exercise, i.e., Good Workout

Let's go and find the best workout for you and me. Let me begin with a conclusion first. In my opinion, the best exercise to maintain and improve our basic health is the exercise of the lower extremities. Of course, the exercise of the upper extremities—chest, abdomen, waist, and back—are important. But the exercise of the thigh muscles should be the most important.

Some people say thigh muscles are the heart that are exposed and that we can see outside. Let's say, the heart in our chest is the invisible heart, and the heart that we can see outside is our thighs. This means that if and when your thighs are strong, your heart is strong. With exercise, when and if you make your thighs strong, your heart will become strong. It does make sense!

Can you catch two birds with one stone? Yes, you can if you are very *lucky*. But you can catch fourteen birds, i.e., small miracles, if you do what I tell you to do. This is exactly what you will be doing and achieving when you exercise your thigh muscles. Maybe more than fourteen if you do what I tell you to do. I'll explain next.

If I claim that I can catch more than ten birds with one stone, not many people would believe me. But I do not mind how many people believe me or not when I tell the truth, as long as I'm telling the truth. I might be alone but will never be lonely because and as long as I stand with the truth.

But there is one thing that bothers me. It's the birds. What are they going to say to one another about me? Are they going to leave me alone? If a person says he can catch or kill fourteen birds with one stone, how would the birds feel? But I do not mind because it is how we express our feeling when we are very lucky. Actually, it has nothing to with the birds per se.

I call these "fourteen small miracles of exercise" when our body becomes alkalotic and subsequently produces endorphin from the pituitary gland, the boss who is in charge of all hormones. It is the control center of all hormones. As a result of a good exercise, our body becomes alkalotic with the help of our two lungs, which is what we call respiratory alkalosis, with which the pituitary gland will produce the amazing hormone, endorphin. Then with exercise itself, along with the effects of alkalosis and endorphin, we shall witness the fourteen small miracles of true exercise in our body.

Here comes formula 2: true exercise = respiratory alkalosis + endorphin (which produce fourteen small miracles).

Numbers 1 and 2, as I mentioned above, with an exercise of the lower extremities, the calf muscles get strong. Then our heart gets strong. The thigh muscles and the heart are twins—one inside, the other outside. If your thighs look strong and healthy, your heart is strong and healthy.

Number 3, our lungs get stronger too. All the indices of lung function improve with exercise, particularly vital capacity. With exercise, the reason we get shortness of breath is not because we have a problem or weakness in the lungs but it is because of the demand coming from the entire body. And with the evidence that our lungs get stronger and of shortness of breath, i.e., hyperventilation, we are developing and moving into the state of respiratory alkalosis.

Number 4, with exercise, blood vessels, especially arteries while repeating constrictions and relaxations, become more flexible. Thus, blood pressure goes down. Currently, we have many wonderful medicines which were not available before. So do not hesitate to take one or two of them. But if you do true exercise, I guarantee your blood pressure will respond better than your meds, and you will be able to cut down the amount and the number of medicines simultaneously. And ultimately, you will be able to control your blood pressure with exercise only. You will be free from medicines and their side effects. What a wonderful life it will be. Just imagine the benefits of true exercise, which I call fourteen small miracles. As result of true exercise, our stable blood pressure will decrease, and we minimize the chance of heart attack, stroke, dementia, etc.

Number 5, with exercise, we increase our carbohydrate metabolism. As a result, our blood sugar drops down. We can control the evil of hyperglycemia with less number of hypoglycemic agents, oral or injectable. Exercise is the best way to reduce high blood glucose, i.e., hyperglycemia, and the best way to control sugar problem, i.e., diabetes mellitus. It is better than diet or pills or injections, etc. If you combine exercise with diet and drug therapy, the success rate of sugar control will be sky-high. If you do not combine it with exercise, the failure rate will go sky-high. There is no need to explain more. How wonderful it would be if we can control high blood sugar without taking sugar pills and without injecting insulin.

Number 6, as mentioned above, blood vessels, especially arteries, become more flexible with exercise. The incidence of heart attacks and stroke goes low, significantly low. Heart attack will not strike you and will go somewhere else. Stroke will not strike you and will go somewhere else too.

Number 7, I already mentioned that cancer also does not like and actually hates an alkalotic environment. I'd like to say that respiratory alkalosis pushes out cancer or kills cancer. This statement is not something that I made up. I'm just quoting what many of the world-famous oncologists, i.e., cancer specialists, are already saying.

Number 8, with exercise, in the blood, bad cholesterol (LDL cholesterol) goes down, and good cholesterol (HDL cholesterol) goes up. This has been proven scientifically a long time ago. What a miracle!

Number 9, if and when we have strong thighs, our back gets strong too. The back pain leaves us, and our old back—strong and young—comes back.

Number 10, if you exercise the lower extremities, not only will the muscles become stronger but also—very important—the joints, such as ankles, knees, and hip joints.

Number 11, when you exercise well, you sleep well too. I'll comment more about this in the chapter "Sleep." Insomnia goes away.

Number 12, if you work out, you will lose weight. I'll comment more about how to lose weight in the chapter "How to Lose Weight: The One and Only and the Best." Also, I'm going to mention about the interrelationship between fat cells, muscle cells, and exercise in the same chapter.

Number 13, if you work out, you will not find the word "indigestion" or "upset stomach" in your dictionary. There is no need to explain. You will have a good appetite and strong stomach as well.

Number 14, as you get older, inevitably, constipation will be one of the many you will end up facing, which you never had when you were young because you are not as active as when you were young. Activity or exercise is the key to avoid this kind of constipation rather than a stool softener. Get up and walk around and work out, instead of taking a stool softener.

There are few more, but I have to cut it short. Because it is getting too long. Just one more thing if I may, workout or exercise is good for dementia, if we control blood pressure with exercise. Let me explain later. I promise.

All the above are scientifically proven. I did not make it up. Why should I? So the conclusion is exercise, exercise, and exercise.

Now we are going to search for good exercise, the true one. What would be the criteria of my true exercise?

First of all, it should not cost you too much. Less money and less time. The cheaper, the better. Causing little to no money would be most ideal. If it costs too much or it takes too much time, it will be eliminated from the category of good workout, such as golf. No matter how good the exercise would be for our body, if it is too expensive and taking too much time to participate, it drops out on my list. Golf itself can be an excellent workout to some people. But not only it is too expensive, it consumes too much time, you cannot do it at night, and so on. You cannot do it if the weather does not help.

Second, the result has to be good. The result? Not only will your muscles get stronger but also what? Didn't I say that there is a problem if an adult goes out and walks for about an hour in his subdivision, comes back home, and says, "Oh, I had a good workout." He might think he had a good workout, but his legs will say, "Not enough!" Do you remember respiratory alkalosis? And endorphin?

Third, it has to be simple and easy to do and safe. It has to be something that you can do under any circumstances or any weather conditions, such as rainy, windy, snowy, stormy, etc. It is something you can do anytime you want, even at night. If it is far away from where you live—such as swimming pools or tennis court, etc.—that it takes too much time to get there, it drops out on my list.

Okay, enough is enough. Let's begin the search! Search for the solution. Since I already recommended lower extremities exercise, particularly hamstring muscles, we are going to think about following four thigh exercises, all of which are excellent workout:

1. cycling
2. jump rope
3. sit-up
4. stairs exercise, the best of all

Before we talk about the above four, let's think about some other excellent exercises, such as tennis and badminton, jogging, walking, hiking, jump rope, etc. These are all excellent thigh exercises.

It is interesting to see weight lifting of any kind. I eliminated weight lifting simply because there is a risk of injury of the back and joints of the upper and lower extremities. There is no question, but we are looking for the best.

Tennis and badminton

These are really excellent thigh muscle exercises. Even though these cost a lot to certain people, compared to the other expensive sports, these are not that expensive.

But the trouble is you have to go to a tennis court to play tennis. It is one of the best sports to build up stamina, tenacity, etc.

You have one more hurdle to overcome. You have to have one or two good partners. But they are human beings too who can get sick in bed or tied up with their business or can go on a vacation like you do. Because we are all human after all.

And another problem is if there is too much discrepancy in the ability between the two players. For one player, it is extreme exercise; for the other, it is no exercise, not even close.

And there is one more serious problem: you can get hurt. Sometimes, you are too slow, or the ball is too fast for you. If you stretch over too much, your ankle, your knee, or your back will inevitably give out. When you are getting older, the healing process slows down. And then if you injure again and again, it will leave a permanent damage. Then you have to give up the one you liked and enjoyed the most. But there is a few exceptions. Somebody I know still plays tennis over the age of seventies and eighties. So it is up to you, but not many can do this.

In the case of badminton, the circumstances are similar.

Walking and jogging, i.e., running

These are also excellent exercises. What a wonderful feeling it is when I walk in the park or run on the trail. Not only I can feel moving into respiratory alkalosis but also endorphin going around my entire body. Yes! These are wonderful exercises. But if you are doing these outdoor, you will face significant limits, such as weather and place.

You need to have a good place to run close to where you are living. But if it is rainy, snowy, or windy, you cannot go out. Due to these limitations, if you join a fitness center, you have to go there to do your favorite workout. To do it indoor, you need a treadmill.

Cycling

This is a really good exercise. One of the best, if not the best. It is exciting! Just thinking about cycling, I feel like I'm flying. It used to be my favorite exercise, but I had to give it up. Let me explain to you why.

First of all, you need to have a good place to ride a bicycle nearby your house, such as parks or schoolyard or subdivision and so on. Otherwise, even if you have a good equipment, it's no use. You have to go outside.

But there will be safety issues because it is not safe sometimes. You can have a minor to serious accident because of not only your fault but also someone else's fault. You cannot go out when the sun is not around. If weather does not help, you cannot do it, no matter how desperately you want to go out.

It is no joke when you are thinking about the cost. The more it looks good to you, the more it will cost you, like when you are buying a car or a house.

As mentioned above, you have to consider the risk of accidents. Because of my mistake as a bike rider, I can hurt myself or others if I am not focused or careful. By the same token, I can get hurt seriously by other's mistake.

Here is another important issue: you need to have a certain level of skills or talents to fix your bike when your equipment breaks down. This was the reason why I had to give up cycling because I have a congenital deficiency in fixing anything.

If you choose indoor bike, you can eliminate many of the above limitations, but you have to make a small sacrifice—a small space of your house or apartment. Sometimes, a stationary bike itself might be too heavy if you want to move it from one place to another in your house or apartment if you do not like the location or, more important, if a furniture or something needs that location.

Otherwise, you have to be a member of a fitness center—meaning, you have to go somewhere from home when you want to.

Sit-up

There is no limitation in this activity. No problem with expenses and no cost for this exercise. You can do it anywhere, and there is no problem with weather at all. So far, so good.

There are so many of advantages compared to others, but the one and only disadvantage of this exercise is that it is so monotonous. It is so boring. But if you do this exercise properly, you will have enormous result. You are going to see enormously strong thigh muscles, which reflect that you have a strong heart.

But I do admit that it is not a good exercise as a primary tool, although it is a good exercise as a secondary tool. I'm sure you will agree.

Jump rope

This is another excellent exercise! I recommend this exercise to as many people as possible in combination with my exercise or other exercises that you prefer.

As you already know, this is a boxer's favorite. When they go into the ring, this is a must. It is so easy and simple, but the result is impossible to describe. When you do it, it only requires a small space. You can do it anywhere, inside or outside. You can do this under any kind of weather. I recommend this exercise highly but as a secondary tool. And with one warning: because there are some people who cannot or should not do this exercise. Someone who has a back problem should not do this exercise, especially in the lumbar spine area, such as lumbar disc diseases, chronic lower back pain, etc. I would say cervical spine too.

If we look at our spine from either side, our spine has a gentle S curve to protect our brain—which is softer than tofu at any grocery store—minimizing the impact coming from below. So the lumbar spine is the one with the curve to protect our brain. The cervical spine is curved also. Then who or what is protecting our lumbar spine? No one. There is no mechanism protecting the lumbar spine. When we jump up and down, our lumbar spine receives more than 90 percent of the impact coming from below. This is the reason why people with back problem should not do this exercise. If you have a low back or neck problem, don't do this exercise. This advice came out of my personal experience. I highly advice you not to do this exercise if you are someone with a back problem. Again, I warned you.

Stairs exercise, the best

Now I'm going to introduce to you the best exercise for our thighs. This is the best exercise of all, in my opinion. Hopefully, it is going to be your best too. I said "the best" because it meets the strict criteria of mine almost perfectly. Again, this is my opinion.

Quickly, let's go over a little disadvantage. You have to be living either in a high-rise apartment building or near one of those. Or you work in a high-rise building.

But if you live in a high-rise apartment or at least taller than a five-story apartment or next to a tall building that is readily and easily accessible, this disadvantage quickly disappears. And there is one small caution: do not run up and down. You have to walk up and walk down slowly. You have to do it slow. You do not need to do it fast, none whatsoever. Surprisingly, it is more effective if you do it slow. The slower, the better!

If you do it fast, only the risk of accidents will go up. To a person who had a bad experience of fall on the floor of a swimming pool or in a sauna, there is no need to explain how bad it is. Particularly, if you are a person who has ankle problem, knee problem, hip problem, or back problem, do it slow, then increase intensity gradually, not the speed but the intensity.

It has nothing to do with exercise itself, but it is good to carry your iPhone while you are doing this exercise. First, there is a stopwatch in iPhone so that you can check your time. Second—this is more important—in case of accident, you can call someone or 911 for help. When you are doing this exercise on the stairs, not many people are doing this exercise; almost always, you will be doing it alone.

This is a true episode about 911. It happened to a family who just moved to the neighborhood of Bloomfield Hills from Korea not too long ago. It was on one December evening when they came back from Christmas shopping. It was a cold and windy winter night. The husband parked his car in the garage and closed the door and started unloading the car. First, he put his children in the bed, then the shopping bags. But one by one, including his wife, started passing out. And finally, the husband himself also started to lose his consciousness. He realized that it was carbon monoxide poisoning, as he remembered that he forgot to turn off his car's engine. This was his first mistake. His second mistake was when he went to the phone, he was dialing 119 instead of 911. At that time, the iPhone was still not in the market. In Korea, the emergency number is 119. Barely he remembered it's 911 in America. Finally, he managed to dial 911, then passed out also. It did not end with tragedy. Because the police responded real quick, no one died. But briefly, the husband was under the suspicion of three first-degree attempted murder by the police. Why did he dial 119 rather than 911? Is there any reason behind? Until they found out that the emergency number in Korea is 119.

Now let's talk about advantages. There are so many. First of all, the cost. You need to buy comfortable shoes and outfit. That is all. That's all you need, and then all you have to do is just go out. Second, since the stairs are located inside the building, it is not affected by any kind of bad weather, such as rainy, snowy, windy, stormy, etc. Weather does not affect you whether you can do it or not. Weather is not an excuse not to do stairs exercise. You can do it even after the sun went to bed. Third, if there is any accident of any kind, you are the one responsible for the accident. You will rarely become a victim of an accident. As long as you do it slow and careful, the chance of accident would be very low. Fourth, if you live in an apartment taller than five floors, where you are going to exercise is in your building. The moment you step out of your door, you can start your workout almost immediately. It is very convenient to do it. There is no travel time to go and come back home, such as in tennis, swimming, etc. You just open your door, and that's already the start of your exercise.

Why five floors? The answer comes very soon. How to do it, and how did I do it? Once upon a time, a famous guru on health issues advised in an article on a newspaper that it would be very good workout if we would go up and down ten floors twice at a time twice a week. So I followed his recommendation and tried exactly the way he said. I failed. I was so disappointed that I failed. It was too hard. I could not finish. It was beyond my ability. I overestimated my ability and could not believe that I was such a loser. I failed after a few trials. I did not realize the simple truth that I had to start from the bottom to climb up to the top of the mountain. So I started from the bottom, not knowing how high the top of the mountain would be. I changed the format entirely. That's how I succeeded by following the simple truth. I went up and down three floors twice at a time, which is a lot less than what the expert was recommending. It was manageable for me. I could see a tiny spot or light at the end of the tunnel. Then I increased the intensity little by little by little. I never ran up and ran down. And then three floors three times at a time. Again, it was manageable and continued for a while. Then little by little, I increased the intensity, filled with confidence that my ability allowed me to do it.

I do not remember the tiny details. I do not remember how long I did. But it became four floors, three times, followed by four floors, four times. Then five floors, four times. Then five floors, five times. Six floors, five times. Six floors, six times. Seven floors, six times. Seven floors, seven times. And eight floors, seven times. Then I could not move up more than nine floors. As a matter of fact, I had to cut down to five floors gradually. Then the number of ups and downs went up to ten times. I tried every which way my body and my ability allowed me to do. I tried more than and less than back and forth to come up with my number. So I do it now five floors ten times ups and downs at a time.

How many times a week? It is a bit simple. I started twice a week initially. Then three times a week and four times a week. Sometimes more than four times a week, almost every day when I feel better or great. Then now it became three times a week. It is every other day and three times a week. It is never like Monday, Tuesday, Wednesday, Thursday, Friday, and Saturday. It is always like Monday, Wednesday, and Friday or Tuesday, Thursday, and Saturday. Every other day.

Now my routine is five floors, ten times at a time, three times a week, which is only a little bit of variation and rarely goes out of norm. And it takes about forty minutes to complete. Forty minutes of excellent workout. For forty minutes, I walk up and down 1,000 stairs. One floor has 18 or 20 stairs. Let's say there are 20 stairs in one floor. Then 20 x 5 floors x 10 = 1,000 stairs. I take 1,000 stairs, taking short breaks when I go up and down each time. So my current numbers are five floors, eight times up and down, and three times a week. That is 583 stairs, in short.

Here is a small piece of advice to those people who are physically handicapped and who cannot do stairs exercise. Even though it might take more time and costs a bit more money, I recommend swimming. Go to a swimming pool. Actually, swimming is the most ideal exercise of all. Exercise in the water and against the water.

We all are made out of water, so we ought to go back to the water. Precisely speaking, our body consists of two-thirds of water and one-third of soil or dust—meaning, one-third will go back to soil, and two-thirds will go back to water. According to the Bible, "Men are from dust, so go back to dust." That has to be one-third correct statement but two-thirds incorrect because our body has two-thirds of water.

Before we were born, we stayed in our mother's "indoor" warm swimming pool for over nine months and were pushed out of the best environment to the harsh reality without our opinion being considered at all. It was 0 percent not our decision and 0 percent not our opinion. We all did come out, but outside was not the most ideal environment. As a matter of fact, we all wanted to stay inside. That's why we were so angry when we were born that we cried all the time.

Anyway, if we go to the sea, river, or swimming pool and jump into the water, we feel like we come home. Exercise in the water is the most ideal and the most effective environment. The best physical therapy of all will be the therapy done in the water and utilizing the gentle resistance of the water. We all came from the water, so we all go back to the water.

So when we are done here and when the moment comes for us to just fade away, we all go back to the water, two-thirds of our body to be exact. And the rest will go back to the dust. As a result, my water meets your water. Then it becomes our water. And our water meets another our water and then becomes a big river and ultimately the ocean in between the big continents. So eventually, we will all meet one another in the middle of the Pacific Ocean.

By the way, from time to time, when I'm in the middle of a strenuous exercise, I experience a strange thing. Sometimes, I do not feel tired. I do not get shortness of breath. I feel very calm. What is happening here? Can I say it is because of endorphin? I'm going to leave the answer up to you.

CHAPTER 4

Rome

I recommend a trip to Europe as many times you can. But if you are a person who tends to focus on one thing or one place, I recommend Rome, Italy.

There is an old saying, "Dig one hole, then you will get a good well that gives you excellent water." As I recommend in the chapter "Travel," you go to Europe in a group setting, visit as many places as you can, then concentrate on one place, and go deeper and deeper as you like more and more.

Rome is the kind of place that the more you visit, the more you will want to visit and see that you have never seen before. Some people who went to Rome as part of a package tour of European countries come back and say, "I went to Rome. I have seen Rome," after spending only two or three days in Rome. In the old days, a wise man asked, "What have you seen in the mountain while on a speeding horse?" It is like, after passing through New York in a speeding race car, claiming, "I have seen New York. Now I know New York." After just licking the outside of a watermelon, what if someone says, "This watermelon is so sweet"? What are you going to say to this person?

There are some, but not many, people who travel to every corner of the world on foot with a minimum cost of money. They work hard, save enough money, then take off. Of course, they study hard about all those places they are planning to visit—geography, history, culture, etc. This is what the so-called travel professionals are doing.

However, majority of us are not travel professionals. So I suggest to the majority, including myself, what most of the people have done so far—set the goal, then work hard, and save money. And when you think that the time has come, take action. These are the same with travel professionals. Then there are millions of different ways of travel packages that are available to us. Take advantage of one of those, once, twice, then become an expert as far as Rome is concerned.

Terminal

I got the impression that it seems like the public transportation of Rome is made not only for the convenience of the citizens of Rome but also of the visitors like us.

"All roads lead to Rome." This was true several thousand years ago in the old Roman Empire and also is true at the present time in the twenty-first century in Rome. You can go anywhere from the terminal and come back to the terminal from anywhere. The terminal is the center of all transportations in Rome from the beginning of the Roman Empire until now and will be forever.

In Rome, there are only two directions where the public transportations are heading—one is to your destination and the other is always back to the terminal. After your day's schedule, for whatever reason, if you choose to take a taxi instead of a bus or a subway train, you just tell the taxi driver "terminal," then he will take you to the familiar place.

If you buy tickets for public transportation, you can use it everywhere and anywhere. The price of the ticket is reasonably cheap, and of course, you can buy a certain amount of tickets at a time so that you do not have to buy every morning. You can carry enough tickets for the day. You do not have to worry if you run out of tickets before the day is over. The trick is simple. You can ride the bus without tickets. Oh yes, you can. The mission of public transportations of Rome is for the safety and convenience of the passengers, not for the money. The bus driver never looks back. He only looks to the front for the safety of his fellow human beings, the citizens of Rome, and, equally as important, visitors like me. The bus driver never looks back to check whether the passengers are dropping the tickets into the box. I'm not encouraging you to take free rides, but when you have no choice, you have to do what you have to. Personally, I'd like to recommend to ride a bus because you can see outside what is going on. The subway train, meanwhile, is convenient and fast to get from one place to another.

So when you visit Rome, it is very convenient if you choose a place close to the terminal, preferably within a walking distance, like within ten minutes or so. When you finished your daily schedule, take a bus or a subway train. Always, you will end up at a familiar place, then just take a walk.

You can find a good restaurant for dinner. Also, you can have a nice-looking bottle of wine, sitting in what looks like a party store or a 7-Eleven in America. One bottle of a decent wine will be good enough for four. Do you remember I prefer to travel with a few, such as two couples? So we have one bottle of a nice and decent-looking Italian wine with dinner for four of nice and decent and happy people.

So you start your day from the terminal and finish your day around the terminal. If you do this as daily routine for a few days, you will already find yourself feeling like you are at home.

Pickpockets

In Rome, if you carry cash or jewelry in your pockets or in your fingers, it is no longer yours.

As a traveler, all you need to carry in your pocket is a small amount of money, enough to buy your lunch and snacks in case you get hungry or thirsty before lunch or before coming back for dinner. You should not carry all your money with you for the entire travel. Always keep all the money at the hotel's safe, and you carry only enough money for the day. All the money you need for one day is for lunch, snack, and drink, like water or pop.

This is not a good subject to talk about, but you have to be careful always if there is any risk to be stolen of your money in order to continue and finish your pleasant trip until you go home. But it is not surprising to see some kind of fallout or negativity, for most of the European countries are the recipients of an enormous number of visitors each year, especially during the peak season of traveling. Most of the European countries are very safe to travel, safer than you think. In general, countries with a large number of visitors have low crime rates, particularly crime rates against travelers.

Another warning or advice if you are planning to visit any foreign country would be not to go out for shopping. Do not waste your time buying things that you can buy here at home in America. Sometimes, you are sure that you bought something from these countries, such as the ones labeled with "made in Italy" in Rome or "made in France" in Paris or "made in Briton" in London, etc. But you will be surprised to find the goods were made in a different country. These items are made in different countries where the minimum wages are very low. You saw the labels clearly—"made in Italy," "made in France," and so on—with your own eyes when you bought the goods. But when you go back to the hotel and look again, the label turned into different countries. I call this "magic." But don't be fooled by this magic or any other magic.

How to Dissect Rome

This is what I do when I go to Italy, specifically Rome. You have to spend at least a day or two to see St. Peter's Cathedral and the Sistine Chapel and then divide Rome by four quadrants and spend at least one or two days on each quadrant.

And if you visit one or two places about one hour or two away from Rome, seven to ten days would be enough. Unlike travel professionals, amateur ones like you and me will get homesick when we stay away from home for more than ten days or two weeks. By then, we are going to miss the comfortable beds of ours waiting for us at home.

Again, once is not enough. I do not know how many times is sufficient to see a place like Rome. That is why, each time you go and see Rome, you say, "I'll be back," like the Terminator. Like anywhere else, if you want to see a place the way it is, you have to study and know the history of the place you are going to visit. This is particularly true when you go to Rome.

I learned the history of Italy and the Roman Empire a bit when I was in high school in world history class. But that is not enough. Not enough to know the interesting parts. We need to know a bit more of the behind story. Then the traveling is going to come to a level of entertainment. We cannot say, "*Veni, vidi, vici*" (I came, I saw, and I conquered) wherever we go and come back.

As you can imagine, there is a big difference between a person traveling with the significant knowledge of history of the area or the country and someone without. The person with knowledge will come back home with much more knowledge about the place than ever before. One person might say, "I came, I saw, and I took pictures." But the other person will say, "I came, I saw, and I learned" and becomes a better person than before.

After traveling, one person remains the same, or worse because they got older. And another person becomes more mature, wiser, and more knowledgeable than before, although this person got older. This is the difference.

History of the Roman Empire

In the beginning, Rome (Roma) was founded in 753 BC. Two countries—ruled by the twin brothers, Romulus and Remus—were united by Romulus. Still, it was a small country that no one or no country paid any attention to.

At that time, Egypt was going downhill, but as a country, Egypt was still powerful while Greece was becoming a powerful country both militarily and intellectually.

And right above, on the north of Rome, there was Etruria, a country with strong military and very skillful people who can build good bridges and roads. We now understand that the Roman Empire army were not only good soldiers in the battlefield but also were very good at building infrastructures, such as bridges, roads, and libraries, etc. Down below, on the south, there were many cities ran by Greeks, who were good at trading by the sea.

Now Carthage (Carthāgo), the scariest country to the people of Rome and may be a stronger and rich country in northern Africa in the area of present-day Libya and Algeria, was always ready to invade the Italian Peninsula. Many times, they came and occupied Sicily, then invaded different parts of mainland Italy. Just looking back to history, Carthage was, indeed, the worst enemy the Roman Empire ever faced.

Rome was located in the middle portion of the Italian Peninsula on the Mediterranean side. The Romans were surrounded by strong enemies everywhere near and far. Not like the Egyptians, the Romans were surrounded by mean and strong enemies everywhere. But sooner or later, the Romans were becoming stronger by conquering or absorbing villages and small countries one by one and building up strength.

Although there must be more than hundreds of reasons why Rome became such a strong and powerful country, it is probably due to the immigration policy it applied to those countries it conquered that it became even stronger by implementing the most successful immigration policy in the history of mankind.

When the Romans engaged in war and won, then the prisoners were given two choices by the commanding general—one was immediate execution or being sold as slaves and the other was Roman citizenship. It was very simple. Depending on the circumstances, it was the commanding general who decided the fate of the prisoners, whether to execute all the captured or to give them the choice to become Roman citizens. Once they became citizens, there was no discrimination, none whatsoever, based on race, religious belief, etc. So in the history of the Roman Empire, they had an emperor of Arabic origin and African origin. That is only if the person is a citizen of Rome.

The worst case of execution by the Romans against any enemy is destruction of everything and execution of everyone as done in Carthage, then Jerusalem. Once the commanding general decided total destruction, then nothing would survive. Nothing means nothing. One example, and the worst of all, is when they won the war against Carthage. They executed every living thing inside the city—all the people, men and women, young and old, even babies, including animals—destroyed everything standing straight to the ground, and then burned everything, whether it was a big city or a small village. So Carthage was burned in three days and three nights. In the end, they dumped a large amount of salt everywhere so that nothing could ever grow out of the ground.

That is the reason why Jesus was weeping out loud, even though all his disciples were watching and listening while he was looking at Jerusalem, where the Holy Temple was, a few days before he died. Apparently, he knew what was going to happen to the Holy Temple by the Imperial Roman army in the near future. Jesus must have seen or knew that, about fifty-some years later, the Holy Temple would be destroyed and demolished by the Romans, as it happened to Carthage a long time ago.

According to the record, there were a lot of people in Jerusalem who came from other countries far and near for the Passover. This episode teaches us that Jesus was one of us. He had all the same emotions that we have—angry, upset, frustrated, crying, and yelling, etc. At the same time, he has the ability to see exactly what would happen in the future. He can see the future as it happens. Meanwhile, we—you and I—have absolutely no ability or no idea whatsoever to foresee who will win in next election, whether and when Dow Jones will have another Black Friday, and so on.

When I go to bed tonight, I have no idea whatsoever whether I'm going to wake up tomorrow morning. So Jesus has the superpower that I do not have. Definitely, he is not an ordinary person like you or me. We have no choice but to admit that he is different, unique, and above us.

After the standoff, almost six hundred thousand people died, and ninety thousand were captured and sold as slaves. Then there happened the total destruction of the Holy Temple and the city of Jerusalem. Many died of starvation, due to shortage of food, or communicable diseases, due to total lack of hygiene because the standoff lasted more than five months.

It is not surprising for Jesus, who knew how much his people were going to suffer, to cry out in spite of his disciples and his followers watching him on his side or behind, who had no idea why he was crying like a baby. He could not control his emotion at all, for only he knew what exactly was going to happen to his people and the temple and his country.

Why did the Jews and Romans hate each other that much? Of course, the Romans were the conquerors, and the Jews were the occupied and conquered. So it is quite natural that the occupied hate the conqueror. But why did the Romans hate the Jews?

Let's consider some other potential factors other than the have and the have-not. Yes, the Romans had everything, and the Jews had nothing. But the Romans knew very well that the Jews were not paying taxes to the Roman Empire. Instead, they sent their money to Jerusalem, specifically to the Holy Temple. And the Jews refused to serve mandatory military service that every citizen of the Roman Empire was proud to do. Last, at that time, the Jews, especially in Rome, were known to get together every night at a secret place and pray to their God, asking his Son to come back again as soon as possible and destroy the Roman Empire with his Father's army from heaven.

His Son Jesus told his disciples that he would die in a cross but would rise from the dead in three days and would then go to heaven to see his Father to report that he completed his mission. Then he would be back as soon as possible. He never told anyone exactly how soon though. So one of his disciples did his best asking him exactly when he would be back but failed to get the right answer we desperately seek because Jesus told him that he did not know when. The disciple took the answer the only way he wanted to hear. His answer was "I do not know. No one knows. Only my Father knows." But the disciple made a huge mistake and failed to remind Jesus that Jesus himself told everyone, including his disciples and his followers, "I know everything that my Father knows."

Absolutely, "I do not know when" is not the answer we are looking for, and he lied. Or at least, it is far from the truth. If not, he did not tell the truth to his disciple. Actually, he himself knew exactly when he will return and even knew how. Even though he clearly knew the answer, he did not want to respond with either yes or no. His answer was "I do not know." It was a lie then and is still a lie now. He did not tell the truth. So that, what all of us—then and now and maybe until the end of our world—are doing is waiting, guessing, and praying like the Christians two thousand years ago inside dark catacombs. If his intention was to make us pray, he succeeded completely. Maybe more than he intended.

Because of this ambiguous answer, all his people did was took it the way they wanted to hear. Of course, if they knew we are still waiting for him to come back even in the twenty-first century and counting, the questioner's and their attitude would have been drastically and entirely different. Certainly, they thought he will be back soon, soon enough that they were still alive in the world. The desperate Jews were asking God to send his Son and his army back to the world and destroy and wipe out the evil empire—exactly what the Imperial Roman army did to their Holy Temple and holy city—and build his eternal kingdom.

We all know that he is not here yet and still do not know when. It was their problem then two thousand years ago. Now it is our problem. Still, no one knows when. No one knows when he will come back. This question became our biggest problem because perhaps somebody was not persistent enough to get the exact answer we want to hear, which is the exact date and time when he will be back. This is the biggest negligence and malpractice at worst and mystery at best of all kind in the history of humanity then and now and perhaps forever. I sincerely hope it is not forever.

Anyway, that was how the Romans punished any enemy of the Roman Empire. They demanded absolute loyalty from the enemy. Or else, there would be complete destruction.

When they won the war against Etruria, they became even stronger—strong enough to get the attention of Carthage, especially by Hannibal and, of course, his father. Hannibal inherited his father's fury against the Roman Empire. The Romans had to go through two gruesome long wars against Carthage—the First Punic War for over 40 years and then the Second Punic War for over 20 years, which was particularly against Hannibal, the best of the best field generals. It took almost 120 long years of struggle, the First and the Second Punic wars combined.

In the history of mankind, Hannibal is the best of the field leaders; no one is better than him. Some people say Alexander the Great should be the greatest. To some extent, I agree. Some might say Julius Caesar should be the greatest field general. Again, I agree. But Caesar is more or less a great politician than a field leader. He might be a great lover too. So Caesar drops to third or below third.

Now between Hannibal and Alexander, who is the number 1? But let's think about their opponents—Hannibal's and Alexander's. Who were their enemies? Though Alexander's opponents were the entire world, they were all amateurs, ordinary person like you or me, not soldiers. On the other hand, Hannibal had one opponent, the Imperial Roman army, which was stronger than the entire world, the war machine, the war professionals, the killing machines. He almost won the war single-handedly against the Imperial Roman army. What a remarkable achievement. I do not mind other people's opinion. But in my opinion, Hannibal is the one and only and the best. And on my list, Alexander the Great would be the second best, a very close second unfortunately.

After the First Punic War (264 to 241 BC), here came Hannibal. He inherited his father's will and anger, which is destruction of the Roman Empire. He wanted to attack the Romans directly by crossing the Mediterranean Sea, but unfortunately, the Romans had a better and stronger navy. The Romans mobilized every single ship they had so that Hannibal could not land on mainland Italy from the sea. Only if Hannibal were able to land in the middle of the Italian Peninsula by the sea—as General McArthur did in the Korean Peninsula during the Korean War—the Roman Empire must have been destroyed and wiped out a long time ago by Hannibal, and the history of the world would have been whole a lot different or entirely different. So he had to go to Spain first and then to Southern France and then cross the Alps then attack Northern Italy.

Victory after victory, he almost took over Rome but just passed by Rome and kept on moving to Southern Italy. No one knows why he did not attack the city of Rome, the heart of the Roman Empire. He had seen the city of Rome from a distance. But he never attacked Rome. Why? He had the ability, the power, and the strength to destroy Rome. Why not? No one knows why not.

The Second Punic War (219 to 201 BC), also called "the Hannibal War" by the Romans, also ended with the Romans' victory. Hannibal died in 183 BC. Carthage disappeared from the earth in 146 BC and became one of the colonies of the Roman Empire. You know the rest of the story.

After the demise of Carthage, the Roman Empire became even stronger, bigger, and more powerful than ever. They expanded and occupied the entire Europe, west of river Rheine, northern Africa, and part of the Middle East and built up the biggest empire in human history. They became the center of the world. Geographically, when we divide Europe between west and east, the benchmark is Rome. When we divide the world between west and east, the same standard is applied. For example, Asia is east, and America is west. China, Japan, and Korea are all east because they are located east of Rome. And Middle East is middle east because it is located in between Rome and east.

Like a human body that gets old with time, the Roman Empire gets old too. They cannot fool aging. Even the Roman Empire cannot avoid the aging processes, i.e., degenerative changes. But the everlasting impact of the Roman Empire will remain with us and will never go away as long as human history continues. Becoming old and senile, Rome eventually split into two empires, west and east (AD 396). Then the west went down first (AD 476), but the east lasted a thousand more years and then disappeared from history (AD 1453). There was no more Roman Empire.

But even after the fall of the Roman Empire, the influence and impact of the Roman Empire continues until now and maybe forever. Even now, we cannot look at anywhere without seeing its influences, such as in politics, military, religion, art, architecture, science, mathematics, diplomacy, immigration policy, sports, transportation, postal service, etc. Its influence is everywhere and everlasting.

That is the reason why we have to go and see what the Romans, i.e., Italy, have done to our lives in the twenty-first century. Although destroyed and divided, with the help of Germany, they led the mainstream of the Renaissance and the awakening of humanity, which is ultimately humanism to the level of what we have now.

Especially in the religious world, humans became the center of religious belief rather than the church. Of course, at the beginning of the Catholic Church, the religion, i.e., the church, was at the center, and people were under the church. It was not too long ago that even reading and owning a Bible was controlled and censored by the church, which had changed long ago.

It was not too long ago, up until the late twentieth centuries, that the spoken language in mass was Latin, which is a dead language long ago—meaning, only priests understood what is spoken, but the people did not understand what the hell was being spoken, which was changed not too long ago.

It was not too long ago that the priest during the mass was standing toward the cross—meaning, people were looking at his back instead of his front, i.e., his face. Now the priest is looking at the people. It was changed not too long ago also.

Gradually but surely, through the teaching of Christ, with the influence of the Roman Empire and the help of the Renaissance and humanism from a church-centered and church-oriented religion, humans moved into and became the center of the religion we have, i.e., Christianity. The Christianity that we believe is human oriented and human centered, not church oriented or church centered. Of course, although we came a long way, we have a long way ahead of us. God resides inside each human heart and exists in the middle of each one of us. That's why we, the people, are the most important of all because Jesus told his disciples and us that we are the most precious and important creation of his Father, who also gave us free will. It didn't take very long for God to realize that the relationship between him and humans took a nosedive from bad to worse because of this free will that was given to humans by him.

At the beginning of Genesis, no sooner than he realized what was happening, God gave humans another important thing called "responsibility," i.e., consequence. That's what we got from God the moment we were kicked out of the so-called garden of Eden. Actually, God gave advanced warning that there would be consequences if humans eat the fruit of the tree of the knowledge of good and evil. When he punished Adam and Eve, he gave specific punishment, i.e., responsibilities, to the man and woman as he promised. But if you look at the punishment closely and carefully, you will find that inside of the so-called punishment, i.e., consequences, he gave humans profound blessings at the same time.

As we grow older, as much as we think we are being punished, we realize that we are given more blessings by him while we are going through what we think to be the punishment of God. It is your homework to figure out what kind of blessings he gave to Adam and Eve, ultimately to us, you and me, i.e., all humans, when he kicked out his most precious creations from his home, i.e., our home.

So humans were given the free will to do anything or everything in this world, but at the same time, it comes with responsibility, also known as consequences, when humans do anything. Like any other things in our life, we are free to choose the good or the bad. When good thing happens after we chose good, we take all the credit. When bad thing happens after we chose evil, we can blame God, but we face the consequences. So it is very fair to God and humans as well.

But there is one thing very interesting: even after we made the bad choice, we are free to think that we made the good choice. Sometimes or many times, even if we commit a serious sin, we are living well and can live as if we did not commit any sin at all. If we make a bad choice, even though we think we made a good choice, we will end up paying the price of making the bad choice in three different timings—immediately, at the end, or in between. The result, the consequence, will come to us regardless of what we think or want—if not sooner in this world, then later when we have to face him in the next world. Only God knows exactly when it is going to happen. As mentioned, in terms of timing of consequences, i.e., the judgment, there are three different timings—immediate, final, and intermediate.

First, as immediate judgment, the best example should be the incident in Genesis. No sooner than they took the fruit, almost immediately, they were kicked out of Eden. Actually, in this episode, there are few things we have to think.

Number 1, the Bible says it was the serpent who made the woman take the fruit. Then how? My question is "How? Was the serpent able to talk?" As far as I know, only God and humans were able to talk. There is no evidence that God gave other animals the ability to talk. Only God and the two humans had the ability to talk. Then it is impossible for the serpent to talk Eve into doing such a bad thing. The person who wrote the Genesis must have had a serious problem with snakes. Some people might say this is a symbolic expression, but I do not accept that excuse.

Number 2, what concerns me the most in this happening is the pathetic and disappointing behavior of the man. When the woman was questioned first, she lied. But the man made two serious mistakes that we should avoid at all costs at the moment we are being judged, which is lying and blaming others for his fault, i.e., sin. When he was questioned why he was hiding behind the bushes, he did two things, which was a huge mistake, at the same time. Based on his response, in my opinion, he was the one who ate first, not second as we assume. Or they, the first couple, discussed and agreed to eat the fruit together, like couples do all the time, if not most of the time. We do this all the time, even when we decide on small things, like what food to eat or which restaurant to go for dinner. We discuss, decide, and then take action. We do this all the time. When he was questioned, he should have said, "I'm the one who ate first. She did it because I told her to. Leave her alone. I'll take the full responsibility." He did something as bad as lying or maybe worse than lying. He blamed his partner for his responsibility, i.e., his mistake. Yes, what's important at this point is, instead of pointing finger at others, that we have to learn a valuable lesson by being honest and taking responsibility for our mistake, especially at the time of the final judgment. As far as I'm concerned, the snake has nothing to do with the incident in Genesis. Leave the snake alone, as it did not or could not talk and could not defend itself. What's important is the fact that they are the ones who decided to eat the fruit. It is not important who ate first or who lured them to eat. Again, what is important is they made the decision to eat and then the behavior of the two afterward in front of God, who was questioning. Leave the serpent alone. It does not know how to talk. Period!

Second, the final judgment. After we fade away, we all go somewhere and have an individual final judgment. That's when we have to remember what happened in Genesis as written above. We should not lie and blame others for our own mistake or sin. We might still be in Eden if the man, whom God created, was honest and responsible.

Third, intermediate judgment. If not immediate, sometimes the judgment will occur anytime in between before the final judgment when we die. The attitude has to be the same as in immediate and final as well. Never relax when you did something bad knowingly or unknowingly and nothing happens; the final judgment is waiting. Intermediate judgment can be skipped if you are lucky. But don't forget the final judgment. That is another advantage of being God. In other words, it is a disadvantage for us.

Between God and humans, I cannot think of any advantages as humans other than free will, which was given by God in the beginning. Yes, he is the Creator of the entire universe. And he made us to be the boss of this world, and then God is looking at the other side. Yes, we are in charge of this world. How good the good God is.

But there are people, countries, or religious groups who do not take advantage of this God-given gift, free will, for the good cause of our side. These group of people or religions are reading their Bible or scriptures and following exactly as written. They read and act based on as written. Nothing in between. No free will in between. No interpretation whatsoever but read and act. They do not allow anything that comes in between. They think it is insulting their God and their belief if anyone makes any attempt to interpret God's intention or negotiate with God or put free will in between God and people. Most of the time, they like to read the way it was written and follow exactly what their founder said, rather than determine what their founder's intention and how their founder acted. There is no interpretation, no questions, no humanity, no human factor, no free will to be settled in their action. They act based on what they see and what is written.

We often see the good example of this behavior when we read the Book of John, chapter 14, where Jesus said, "I am the way, and the truth, and the life. No one comes to the Father except through me." What did he mean by this? Do we have to believe the way it is written? Or have we thought twice or more if necessary?

According to the way it is written, if this is true, only Christians are in heaven, no one else. But in my opinion, there are many non-Christians who are in heaven too. Many Christians will be angry at me if I dare say that there are more non-Christians than Christians in heaven. My answer is no one knows. Have you been in heaven? Have you seen it? Let's leave this conclusion until we meet again in heaven.

As a matter of fact, I wrote the answer on the last page of this book. It starts like this way. There was a Christian who went to heaven when he died. The person was so surprised and shocked three times when they went inside.

As humans, Jesus showed us the best example of free will that was given to us and how to use it by what he did the night before he was crucified. He asked not his Father's intention, the reason, or the purpose of what will happen tomorrow. All of them he knew so well already. He asked the most desperate request that anyone would ever make with free will. Of course, I assume he asked his Father the purpose of tomorrow already, but he knew the answer so well too. It is no time to ask that question why he had to be crucified. Why would the Son of God have to die for no other reason than the will of his Father? Only because it's the will of his Father. The time to ask his Father's plan or intention had passed a long time ago. But still, he did his best and asked his Father to make it not happen what was going to happen the next day. He used his free will to the best of his benefit by asking his Father to erase the tomorrow's event from the calendar. But almost immediately, even before his Father answered him, he told his Father to do it as he planned.

This is what we have to do with our free will—do our best by asking God whatever questions we have to our own benefit. Who knows if he listens and changes his mind and does something good for us. We are free to ask any desperate questions of ours to the Father of Jesus Christ, who is our Father as well.

Most of the times, we know the answer even before we ask the question, like Jesus did two thousand years ago. But if we do not know the answer, we should just keep asking for the answer until God gives it to us or until he gives up. Who knows? Again, how good the good God is for giving us free will. And for giving us a chance to interpret his intention and ask for the answer for our own benefit.

While I was studying the history of the Roman Empire, my curiosity would take me to the history of Greece and furthermore to the history of Egypt. That is why I left my small footprints as much as I could in Abu Simbel in Egypt. Of course, the founder of Christianity was born in Judea, then the colony of the Roman Empire. And to avoid persecution of the Roman Empire, he went to and grew up in Cairo, Egypt, for more than a few years. When you go to Cairo, you will visit the village where Jesus grew up with his parents.

After the crucifixion of Jesus and after the total destruction of the Holy Temple, Christians escaped to Rome, the center of the world, and spread the good news like a wildfire from the ghetto of Rome to the entire Europe and to the rest of the world with help of the Roman road, that was constructed by the soldiers of the Imperial Roman army. How ironic it would be. The Imperial Roman army demolished the Holy Temple of Jerusalem. Christianity spreads to the world with help of the Roman road built by the same soldiers of the Imperial Roman army who destroyed Jerusalem. How ironic it is. "And you know the rest of the story. And have a good day!"

"Have a good day!" was a famous line by Paul Harvey. Now he is gone, but he was a famous radio personality in Chicago, whose morning show was heard everywhere in this part of the country. I could hear his unique voice every morning on the way to my work. At the end of his program, he used to talk about an interesting and unusual story, an incident, an event, or an accident that happened recently or a long time ago without telling the person's name in his story. Then at the end, he finished his morning show by spitting out the person's name and saying in his unique way, "And you know the rest of the story. This is Paul Harvey. Have a good day!" After making his audiences curious the entire time, he finished the story abruptly. By the time his listeners realized what is the true meaning of his stories, he was long gone already.

When you are traveling Europe or Italy, more specifically Rome, I recommend you to choose the timing during the off-season. If you travel Rome in peak season, such as in summertime, the entire Europe is on vacation, which means it is a nightmare for all the travelers. First of all, avoid the winter season. You have to walk around, sometimes stand outside in a line, waiting a long time to buy tickets and get in and so on. It is cold outside. It is not good traveling in winter. And during spring break, summer vacation, or fall recess, there are too many travelers you will be wasting most of your valuable time waiting on the line, looking at the person's head and behind in front of you rather than watching famous paintings or sculptures. So I recommend the off-season, like from mid-February till mid-March. Again, you have to decide when to travel based on your personal schedule. The period I'm recommending is still cold, but not winter cold. It can be cold when the sun goes down, but when the sun is up and out, it is comfortable outside. You are going to need the kind of clothes which is very warm and comfortable and light. Lightness is very important to minimize the weight you carry. To satisfy those difficult requirements, I usually go to Costco and do my shopping.

Vatican

Now we go to Vatican.

It takes approximately thirty to forty minutes from the terminal to Vatican if you take a subway. So you start early in the morning. Then you have to do the thing you do the most at the entrance all the time while traveling—waiting in line.

There was a long line. We waited for about forty minutes to get the ticket and went inside. During the peak season, the waiting would be minimally two hours according to the tour guide.

When you go inside, go to the Vatican Museums and see the David statue and other famous collections but do not spare too much time in the museums because there is a whole a lot of things to look that are waiting for you.

Sistine Chapel

It is small chapel attached to St. Peter's Cathedral. It was built as the pope's personal chapel. In 1477, Pope Sixtus IV restored the chapel and named the chapel after himself.

Then between 1508 and 1512, during Pope Julius, Michelangelo painted the famous ceiling. But because of the famous paintings on the ceiling and the walls depicting the Genesis of the Old Testament, it is as famous as or more famous than any other must-see spots. Also, this chapel is used when the cardinals elect a new pope, also known as a papal conclave.

There is a time limit once you get in, so you have to come out even though you want to stay a bit longer. You have no choice, for other visitors like you. Also, once you get in, you cannot take a picture. You have to print in your brain what you see inside. So this is one of the places that you have to study or research before you come. Though you want to stay longer, you have to come out after a certain time. Your neck will be stiff because everybody, including you, has to look at the ceiling, looking for the painting you want to see, such as the painting of God and Adam trying to reach each other's index fingers, like the boy and E. T. in the *E. T. the Extra-Terrestrial* movie.

In the movie, E. T. touched the boy's bleeding index, showing the healing power. But in the ceiling of the Sistine Chapel, God and Adam are not touching with their index fingers. We do not know what is going on here. The next moment, God touched the human's finger. It's a mystery.

According to my friends who went to the Sistine Chapel way ahead of me, they were able to stay inside as long as they wanted and were able to take pictures as many as they wanted. But now that has changed when I went there.

As far as I can remember, the Sistine Chapel was closed several times—when a new pope has to be elected and when restoration work needed to be done and in progress. I do not recall the exact year, but it was more than twenty years ago, and the chapel was closed for several years.

The Vatican was having a big headache because the Sistine Chapel has such a small space, and yet so many people have been in and out of it for so many years. The paintings on the ceiling and wall show signs of contaminations by human sweats, perfumes, cigarette smoke, body odor, etc. The Vatican decided to do a major restoration on the Sistine Chapel. Initially, the Vatican wanted a group of Italian experts to take care of the restoration, but the expense was so astronomical that they had to look at somewhere else. When they contacted Japanese experts, they were given an offer that they could not refuse. The Japanese group told the Vatican that they would complete the work with no charge at all, but with one condition. The only condition in the Japanese plan was that nobody can take a photo of the Sistine Chapel anymore but themselves. The Vatican gave the permission to take photos only to the designated group of experts. The restoration began in 1980 and took ten years.

Naked God

So it was a story of restoration that happened in a recent memory. This story is something that happened at the beginning. After the wall painting was done, the Vatican asked Michelangelo to do the painting of the wall behind the altar and the ceiling. He took the job reluctantly because he considered himself a sculptor, not a painter. While he was painting the ceiling and the wall behind the altar, he did not allow anyone inside, except a few of his apprentices. But it did not take too long that the big secret leaked out to the cardinal who was in charge of the project. He painted God naked. Adam can be naked. Even Jesus can be naked. But it is absolutely unacceptable for God without covering the "thing" in the middle. So the order came from the cardinal to cover that area.

The difficult task was given to and accomplished by one of his apprentices, and the cardinal was given the "honor" of having that painful face of a human who was sent to hell and tortured by demons painted by the painter himself, Michelangelo. If some scientist invents a super eraser, then we might be able to see the "true" God someday.

When we go to the Holy Family church (Basilica de la Sagrada Familia), in Barcelona, Spain, on the top of one of the four entrances, we can see the naked Son of God. We have to watch this sculpture with our neck extended, like we have to see the ceiling. The Son on the cross with arms stretched does not wear clothes, and so his VIP (very important part) is exposed. One thing you notice from the many people looking up and watching is no one, including myself, looks embarrassed about his missing pants.

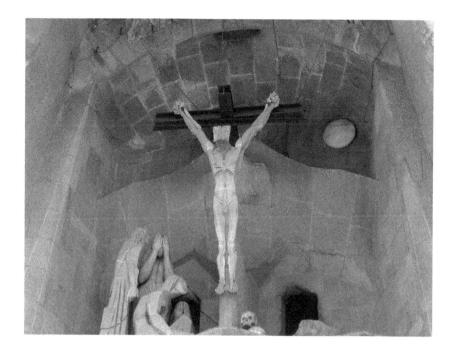

Historically, our ancestors did not wear pants because it was not yet invented or available at the time of more than two thousand years ago. According to the Bible, before he was crucified, all his clothes that he was wearing were taken away by the Roman soldiers. It is correct historically and artistically that the Son should not wear pants.

When you are looking at the Son on the cross who just died but with the pants on, you might be looking at someone else. And yet if you believe he is the One, you are a true believer.

The Pietà

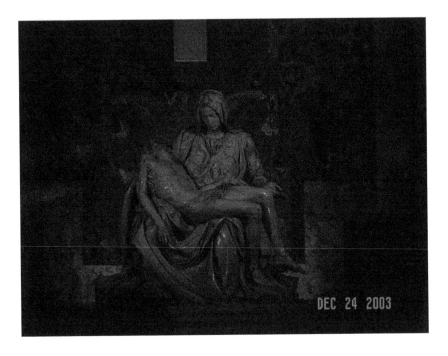

DEC 24 2003

After we were "pushed out" or "kicked out" or, to be more polit-ically correct, told to leave the Sistine Chapel, we went to the top of the St. Peter's Basilica. It is not easy to climb up to the top, but you have to do it at least once to look at the entire Vatican City. Then come back down and find a decent restaurant to have a nice lunch.

Finally, we went into the St. Peter's Basilica. My heart was still racing and pounding due to the electric shock from the ceiling of the Sistine Chapel.

There are so many things to see and talk about inside the basil-ica, but I'm going to talk about one thing, only one thing. I had no idea whatsoever about another far greater shock that I was about to receive from the same person. Again, my poor soul had no idea what was coming. I was totally unprepared. Like any other cathedral, we saw three big doors in the front of the basilica. The middle door is bigger and taller than the two doors on the right and left. The door on the right was shut. I noticed the reason why immediately when

I went inside. So I went through the biggest of the three doors, the middle one. Then when I turned immediately to the right, my heart froze. I do not remember how long. My heart stopped. There she was. With her son on her laps. How many times did I see it in the textbook, magazine, newspapers, and so on? It is true, and I never realized that it is true that "seeing is believing" until I saw this. You have to see it to convince yourself to believe what you are seeing. It is the *Pietà*, sculptured by the same person who painted the ceiling of the Sistine Chapel. Everybody's facial expression looked alike. It seemed all were hit by a lightning.

Oh no, it is like being touched by the gentle hand of the true love of God, who gave us such a loving mother. Not only she is her Son's mother but also she is our mother. There is an old saying, "When the husband dies, the wife buries him on the hill. But when her child dies, the mother buries the child in her heart." This is the moment the mother buries her son in her heart. When we die—no, when we just fade away—she will do the same for us. When I fade away, she will do the same for me. Let's not be afraid when we die—no, when we fade away. There she is, who will bury us in her heart like our own mother. Now we know that we have two amazing ladies who will more than willingly give you and me their warm hearts for us to rest eternally. The entire Christian faith is expressed in this rock. You can feel the entire Bible just by looking at this. Why waste our time? Just go to Rome and simply take a look it. The entire Bible will go to your heart.

This remarkable work was done in 1498, when Michelangelo was twenty-three, only twenty-three. When he finished, this young sculptor himself was so glad to see what he did he could not stay away from it. Every afternoon or evening at the end of the day, before he went home, he would sit down from a distance and watch his masterpiece then go home.

On one afternoon, another happy hour he was enjoying, unintentionally, he listened to some people's conversation to each other, and he noticed the conversation almost becoming an argument. In the beginning of the conversation, he was happy because everybody was unanimously complimenting the sculptor. When the conversation moved to who was the sculptor, no one knew who. They guessed and spit out many names, but his name never came out. He went home furious because no one knew and said his name. When he came back the next day, he brought his tool with him. And he carved his name across the chest of the grieving mother. This is the only sculpture with the sculptor's name on it. If you go and stand close to it, you can see what he did. I'm talking about his name.

I'm not a psychiatrist, but I'm sure he has a personality disorder, an obsessive-compulsive type. Why did he do such a stupid thing? He regretted later what he did and pledged he would never do it again. The answer is because he has an obsessive-compulsive personality disorder, a big-time personality disorder. People with this disorder always regret what they did wrong. Psychotics never regret. Crazy people never apologize.

Insanity versus Personality Disorder

In this world, there are many things that we can imitate but cannot duplicate. If we want to be someone in the past or present, we have to do our best as we can. That is all we can do. There are some things that we can overcome, but at the same time, there are many things that we cannot. We should know that we can pretend to be somebody, but we cannot be that somebody. The only thing we can do is pretend or give up.

We can pretend to be Michael Jordan, but you cannot duplicate what Michael Jordan did. Do you think you can do it? Oh, please don't! Just be yourself. We can pretend to be Wolfgang Amadeus Mozart, but you cannot be Mozart. We can pretend to be Michael Jackson or Elvis Presley, but we can only imitate them. You can pretend to be John F. Kennedy, but I know John Kennedy. You are not John Kennedy. You want to be Leonardo da Vinci, Vincent van Gogh, or Michelangelo? You can imitate them. That's all you can do. But in this case, if you think you can do better than Michelangelo, of course, you are not he. If you think you can do as good as or better than Michelangelo, that means you are suffering from schizophrenia, a paranoid type with grandiose delusion.

It happened in 1972, and the damage was caused by a mentally disturbed Hungarian-born Australian young man, who thought he can do better than or as good as Michelangelo. When he realized he is not him and is far inferior to him and he cannot be him, he went to the St. Peter's Basilica with a hammer. He dealt fifteen blows and thus gave multiple damages to the *Pietà*. He was subdued by the other visitors. Mary's left arm at the elbow was broken. Her nose and few others were broken too. Many pieces were taken by the visitors nearby at the time of the accident. Most of them were returned after a heartfelt request by the Vatican, but some pieces were never returned. Somebody has it at home.

After a careful and meticulous restoration, the *Pietà* is now sitting behind and protected by a bulletproof glass panel, but you may not recognize it because the glass is so well maintained and so clean.

One of the characteristics of a psycho is that they never apologize for what they have done, even after they committed a murder or multiple murder because they think they have done nothing wrong.

Costco

From mid-February to end of March in Rome, it is pretty cold when the sun goes down. You need a jacket which is very light and very warm as well. Of course, the price has to be reasonable or not expensive. When the sun is out, it is like a fall weather. But when the sun disappears, it is really cold and chilly.

A store which meets the above criteria is Costco. There were so many stores like Costco that came and disappeared due to stiff competition, but this one seems to stay with us for quite a long time. Costco's brand name is Kirkland Signature, which means if at certain items they are very excellent in sales, they will produce their own items and sell them at a very reasonable price. This is one of the big differences between Costco and other companies that came and went.

So I'm going to list several more reasons why Costco will remain my favorite store for years to come.

First, it is the people, the employees. The people who are working there look happy or pleasant all the time. When you get in, you are greeted with a smile. When you are leaving, you will see their smiles. If you have any question, you will get the answer with a smile. Most likely, they are being paid more than the employees in other stores. How much more? I do not know.

Second, what is the most favorite fast food that Americans like the most? McDonald's, Burger King, Wendy's, Subway, pizza, what else? All wrong! They put a bait in front of people's mouth that people cannot turn away. The answer is hot dog. None of the above fast-food restaurants sells hot dogs. I do not know the reason why, but maybe it is too easy to make. Many people who are done with shopping eat hot dogs and then go home. Costco makes an excellent hot dog with 100 percent beef. Most hot dogs are not made of 100 percent beef. On top of the quality, the size is big. And then for the bun, they use the top quality of flours. So not only the taste is excellent but also the price is more than reasonable. The current price is $1.50, including all-you-can-drink pop. In the beginning, it must have been just one dollar. Hot dog is the best fast food when you play golf. And when we go to the park for a picnic with families, with other fast foods, we always make sure to bring hot dogs. We also put the so-called chili, which is ground beef, on the top of the hot dog, then additionally boiled American cheese on the top of all those, and then eat it. Nothing can match this taste. And then they added pizza, which is my favorite, and a few others to their menu. Also, this pizza is not a joke. Because they used the best quality of flours and other materials. The taste is excellent, and the price is excellent too. The taste is as good as any other pizza restaurant, and the price is incomparable with other pizzas. With one big piece of pizza alone, it costs you only $1.50. And if you include an all-you-can-drink pop, it is $1.99. It will be just a little over $2.00 with tax. That's all.

And third, when they build a Costco store, it looks like a huge warehouse with plenty of parking spaces. They build a gas station at the corner of the parking area and sell gasoline at the price cheaper than any other gas stations. So the customers who came for shopping put gas on their cars on the way out if the tank is low or empty. You can save $3.00 to $5.00, depending on the size of your gasoline tank.

Finally, just because I spoke so highly of Costco, I did not receive anything or any bribery from the CEO of Kirkland Signature in Seattle, Washington. I have nothing to do with Costco.

Catacombs

There is one more place we need to go. If you go to Rome in a group with a tour guide, you will not be able to see this place. Because this is not a place for tourist attraction. There is nothing artistically valuable or historically important.

There is a small church in a walking distance from the Catacombs of Rome, which is forty or fifty minutes away from the terminal by bus or subway train. The cemetery for the emperors or dignitaries is located inside the city of Rome, but the poor or the deserted are all buried in these catacombs, which became one of the tourist attractions. When you go to the catacombs, just remember this church is in a walking distance. If you have enough time, pay a visit for your own curiosity.

When you go into the labyrinth of the underground tunnel of catacombs, you touch the wall, the stony hard wall, and think, "How this is possible? How is this wall standing? How is this wall still standing?" I do not know the answer. I'm not an engineer or an architect. If you know the answer, share with me.

How big is this underworld? The tour guide said no one knows how big. This is the perfect place for early Christians to have prayer meetings together without being caught by the Roman soldiers. Even the first pope was buried here temporarily after he was crucified, somewhere in the tunnel of the catacombs, then moved to the current burial site, below the altar of the St. Peter's Basilica.

Ordinary Guy Nero

Long, long time ago, in Hollywood, there was an actor who was very handsome and tall, more handsome and taller than Clark Gable. His name is Robert Taylor. One of the memorable movies that he made was *Quo Vadis*.

When Peter recognized his crucified teacher in the early morning darkness, frightened Peter cried out, "*Domine, quo vadis?*" The movie title came from what Peter said out of panic.

In that movie, like many other movies or TV stories, the emotionally unstable Nero set fire to the city of Rome and then blame it to the Christians to avoid the responsibility. In many other movies, including this one, Nero was depicted as a leader, a middle-aged man, and emotionally so unstable that he enjoyed watching the innocent people, the Christians, dying horribly, either burned to death or killed by starved beasts.

He, Nero, was and still is a typical example of what would happen if a person who is intellectually unfit and emotionally unstable becomes the leader of the world or the leader of the Roman Empire. Maybe he was emotionally unstable and intellectually unfit for his position in his later life or after he became emperor. But as far as I know, he was an average guy you can see among your friends or cousins.

Nero was only sixteen years old when he became the emperor of the Roman Empire. And then when he killed himself, afraid of being captured and executed by his own soldiers, he was only twenty-one years old, not even thirty. Actually, he was born to be a perfectly normal, average, and ordinary person. Just like you or me, he liked to sing. He must have had a good or excellent singing voice. He could have won such a competition like *America's Got Talent* or *American Idol* easily by singing his own song. Of course, he composed his own song. Yes, he was a singer and songwriter. He liked to sing his own song. Yes, he got a gold medal in the Olympics in singing contest and then toured Greece with his own band and received a very enthusiastic response from the audiences in Greece.

If he were born in modern-time America, he would have been a singer and songwriter, like John Denver or Bob Dylan, who lived a happy life and made others happy with his songs and would have won a Nobel Prize. But the difference between him and us or John Denver and Bob Dylan happened to be that he had a superintelligent, supersmart, and superenergetic soccer mom as his mother.

As you can imagine, like we have seen it modern times in the twenty-first century, if a leader becomes a leader solely with the help of someone else, then the person or, many times, the people who made him the leader become the leader behind the leader, if the leader is intellectually immature or unfit for the job. So Nero became the leader of the Roman Empire. The empire is not run by the emperor but by the person who made him emperor, to be exact, in Nero's case, his mother.

Anyway, as he grew older, he started feeling threatened by this dominant and domineering mother. He became paranoid about his own mother, which was such an ambitious person that she herself might want to become an emperor or empress someday. What if it was soon? When was it going to be? What if that was tomorrow?

Like any other average person, finally, he made up his mind to eliminate the dominant figure hovering over his head and telling him what to do and not to do all the time. So he took action on her before she could take action on him. He killed his own mother with his own hand, with his sword, by stabbing her.

As you can imagine, if a person is a singer and songwriter, they are an environmentalist. And so is Nero. The city of Rome was flooded with people from all over the world. Even before Nero became emperor, the city of Rome was crowded not only with people but also with bad housing, next to one another and sometimes on the top of one another. There were all kinds of symptoms and signs that Rome was becoming a slum or already became a slum by the time Nero became the emperor. So when there was a fire, it was extremely difficult to put it out. And Nero, the environmentalist, mentioned from time to time that the city of Rome needed to be rebuilt to prevent a disaster from happening. Indeed, there was a fire which went out of control, a big fire that burned the city of Rome for three days and nights. In the movie, Nero was enjoying watching the fire on the top of his palace. But in reality, he was in panic because the fire at that time was too big to handle. The only thing that the citizens of Rome, including the emperor, was able to do was watch the fire burning.

At the same time, a rumor was spreading out to the people much worse than the fire itself, which was that the emperor was the one who set the fire to clean up the dirty city of Rome. Nero was so desperate to do something to defend himself because he was facing two potential disasters simultaneously. For the fire, he had nothing else to do but watch it helplessly like anybody else. For the rumor, someone gave him an idea to put out the fire of rumor instantaneously blame it to the Jews and the Christians. They came to Rome after their leader was executed by his own people. At the time of Nero, the Christians were already the object of an ever-deepening hatred. On the other hand, the Jews refused to serve in the military, like every citizen of the Roman Empire had to do and was doing. The Romans took a great pride in being a soldier of their own country, the Imperial Roman army. The Christians also refused to pay the tax, like every citizen of the Roman Empire had to do and was doing. Christians sent their "tax" to the temple in Jerusalem. They refused to recognize the Roman Empire as their own country. Instead, when they were together, they prayed to their God to send their leader back to earth, who died not too long ago, and establish a new kingdom. So Nero sent out his soldiers and started executing Christians in public.

This was the time, when Peter, the next leader of all Christians, decided to avoid the persecution of the Roman Empire by running away from Rome to save his and his family's life. When his followers got caught on the streets and executed by being burned and being eaten by hungry beasts, he chose to save his own life. So on one night when everybody was fast asleep, he put everything he owned and all his family in a wagon and left Rome. When he was passing a hill nearby the catacombs, it must have been very early in the morning. From Rome to that point, it took forty to fifty minutes in a subway train, but he was on foot. We can safely say that it was very early morning when the sun was about to come out. He might have been thinking whether he should take a break. At that moment, he saw a person coming from the opposite direction. The person was tall like his teacher, but he told himself, "No, no way he is the one." Shaking his head, he added, "He could not be!"

As the distance between the two got closer, Peter recognized immediately who that young man was. Apparently, it was not at night. It was not during the day. If it was in the middle of the night, they would not have recognized each other. They would have passed by each other. Especially Peter would not have recognized because he was in a hurry to save his life. If it was bright daylight, Peter would have recognized his teacher from a distance, run away from him, and hidden where his teacher could not find him. Peter is well-known to us that he ran away from his teacher and hid to save his life more than once. On one single day, he ran away three times when the accusers recognized him. I think Jesus chose the time of morning darkness, not pitch-black or broad daylight. Otherwise, the meeting between the two would not have occurred. The most important meeting ever in the history of Christianity would not have happened.

That is why timing is everything in our lives. Momentum is so important. When the two came so close to each other, almost face-to-face, they recognized each other. As usual, out of panic, Peter cried out, "*Domine, quo vadis?*" He did not ask who he was first, why he was here, or where he came from. Out of all those many questions, he was more concerned about the direction more than anything. "Where are you going?" is "*Quo vadis?*" Out of free will and out of nowhere, Peter chose this question, the most important and famous question in the history of Christianity, without thinking.

Just imagine if this meeting had not occurred, modern-day Christianity might not be existing. Then what about you and me? We do not know how long they talked to each other. But we do know the rest of the story.

There is a small church not far from the road where they met on that early morning, although we do not know the exact spot. The road where they met was built by the emperor Appius Claudius Caecus in 312 BC, one of the roads leading to Rome. In Latin, the name is *Via Appia Antica*; in Italian, *Via Appia*; and in English, the Appian Way. This road is also famous, and of course, Hollywood made a movie with it named *Spartacus* (111 to 71 BC).

When Spartacus revolted against the Roman Empire, even though he was gaining victory after victory, he knew he could not defeat the Imperial Roman army in the long run. He made a careful escape plan. He made a deal with the owner of many commercial ships to escape to far, far away across the sea, a place where the Roman soldiers could not find them. But the deal was broken off by the shipowner, who was afraid of a stiff retaliation by the Romans.

Spartacus died in the battle near the Appian Way, and those who were captured were brought to this road. Thousands of the captured were executed by crucifixion on crosses lined up on both sides of the road. Spartacus died in 71 BC at the age of forty. By the time, his countless men died on the cross, the cruelest way to punish those who betrayed the Roman Empire. If you know you are going to be crucified, you would rather choose to die in battle. Just imagine how humiliating it would be when every passerby is watching you on a cross, dying with no cloth on.

Almost one hundred years later, at the age of thirty-three or so, Jesus also died on a cross with no cloth on, exactly the same way Spartacus's men died, in front of his own mother.

On that road, the Appian Way, there is a small church that is not fancy and definitely not a tourist attraction. But if you choose to go inside, you will see a pair of footprints on a marble stone, which was said to be the footprints of Jesus that appeared after the incident of the famous meeting. But did anyone see when it happened? Nobody had an iPhone for sure. It is a copy; the original is kept somewhere else.

I'd like to ask a small question, which is "Why are we waiting for the second coming of Jesus Christ?" Is it not the third coming that we are waiting? Because he made his second visit already to this world—to be exact, to Peter—the most crucial meeting between Jesus and the first pope. It does not count because it is unofficial, and there was no one who saw their meeting.

On every Christmas, when we celebrate the birth of Jesus, why are we told that we are waiting for the second coming of Jesus? In my opinion, it has to be the third. We all are waiting for his third coming or visit. What do you think?

CHAPTER 5

Water

Let me begin with the definition of the best water for our body. Luckily, we have good water all around us. But no one or almost no one knows how to make a good and ordinary water into the best water for our body. Certainly, the quality has to be good, clean, and uncontaminated chemically and biologically, etc.

We are lucky enough to have good water around us, especially in Michigan, which is right next to the Great Lakes. We are so fortunate. But in this world, there are many countries and many people who have no choice but to drink less-than-good water. It is very important to have good water first. And then we have to make this good water the best water for our body if possible. That is the main goal of this chapter.

I do not have any magical power to turn less-than-good water into good and then into the best water. All I can do is to make the good water into the best. Yes, this is my magic. From good to the best. I must have a good water to begin with though. In this chapter, the main issue that I want to talk about is how to make a good water the best water. This is how.

Like any other things in our lives, making the best from the good also depends on timing. The timing has to be good. Timing is the key. This is my magic. Timing, timing, and timing is my magic.

The best water in this world is the water that I drink when all the cells of my body needed it the most. The plain water next to me when my body needs it the most—which is when my cells are thirsty, i.e., dehydrated, not my tongue or my lips—is the best water. Why not when I feel thirsty? I drink when I feel thirsty. Wrong! Dead wrong! Because it is too late. This is why.

By the time you feel thirsty in your mouth or in your brain, your cells are already dehydrated, which means you are opening and entering the doorstep of death of your cells—plain and simple. By the time you feel thirsty, by the time your lips and your tongue feel dry, it is already too late. That's why timing is so important. Of course, the quality of the water is important. At the same time, timing is also important. If our government, our society, or our community provides good water, then we must focus on the timing.

So in order to make good water the best, we need timing. Like anything else in our lives, timing is the key. You have to drink water before you feel thirsty. This is the key. Most of us are looking for a good water, and most of us do have a good water. From now on, we have to learn and train ourselves to make the good to the best. However, we cannot look inside our body. Specifically, we cannot put our cells under a microscope. There is no other way to tell when our cells need water. We cannot put a microscope into our body.

So unlike any other chapters, in this chapter, let me tell you the conclusion first, which is drink water wisely. It means drink a little and drink frequently before we feel thirsty. We are in trouble if we drink too little. Or if we drink too much, we are in trouble too. The only and the best way to drink water is little and frequent.

The water content of our body is a bit over two-thirds, which is up to 70 percent. And only one-third or 30 percent is not water. That means if a person is weighing 150 pounds, only 50 pounds is not water—meaning, 100 pounds is water. Just imagine how much water we are dealing with if a person is weighing over 300 pounds.

So to be exact, when we fade away, majority of our body has to go back to water, not dust. Water is two-thirds in amount, almost twice the amount of the dust. Only a small portion of our body goes back to dust. It is more accurate when we say "from water to water" rather than "from dust to dust." We go back to the water more than to the dust, more than twice the amount of the dust, to be exact.

Most likely when God found out that his most precious creation, i.e., man, disobeyed him and took the fruit of the tree of knowledge of good and bad without consulting him, he must have been so upset, angry, and confused that he forgot to mention the fact that he made man out of two-thirds water and one-third dust to be exact, more water than dust, twice as much. He said in Genesis, "For you are dust, and to dust you will return." He forgot to mention the most important element of his own creation, water. So this portion of the Bible has to be rewritten. You know what has to be done.

Evidently, the dust part of our human body is the one that makes us unique and different from one another, and the water part of us is the one that makes us sharing similarity and identity among ourselves. And it is not surprising that we see in God's creation of man that we share more similarities than differences among ourselves. When we look at one another, we have to try to see water than dust. We try to recognize our similarities rather than the differences. This is why we see more similarities than differences in ourselves, and this is what we have to do to find more similarities than differences in ourselves. God created all of us equal and more similar than different from one another.

To achieve this goal to reach the goal line, we are already past more than half of the length to the finish line. We are at a seventy-yard line on a one-hundred-yard dash. Which one is easier to achieve—finish the thirty yards or go back the seventy yards? Hey, America, we came a long way to recognize the similarities in ourselves. We see the finish line right in front of our own eyes. The entire world is watching us. Just take a few more steps! Don't turn around. Don't go back to where we started.

It is your homework to calculate where you are and how many miles you have to go. We have only less than 30-some percent to achieve. Isn't that nice? I hope everybody moves forward and finishes the less distance rather than turn around and go back the more distance. Which one does our God want us to choose? Or which one do you want to choose? You have the answer in your heart already. I hope you have the same answer I have. We came a long way to realize we are all created equal

Water is so important to our body. We will all fight for drinking water in the future rather than oil. Actually, it is already happening inside the US, not far from us. I live in Michigan, near the Great Lakes, where we do not hear much about water shortage or drought and so on. But many states, like California, Nevada, Arizona, Texas, etc., are going through serious water shortage every year. Sometimes they request assistance, but the governors of the Great Lakes decline each time. Even the federal government or the president of the USA cannot order these states to share the water. A silent war is already going on inside the US, not to mention outside of it. In my experience, the water from the Great Lakes is better than any water among all the good waters of the entire world.

And deep in the Canadian Rocky Mountains, we can have a rare opportunity to see a glacier ice water. Over thousands of years, tens of thousands of years, hundred thousands of years, or millions of years ago, heavy snow after heavy snow, accumulation after accumulation, all the snows turned into glacier and, then over the glacier, another one and another one and another one. Due to the weight and the gravity, the giant glacier is pushed down little by little. When it is pushed down to a certain level to hit the temperature of melting point, the glacier starts melting. And it forms a small creek on the top of the glaciers. If you put your hand in this creek, you will lose the feeling of your hand within a few seconds. When I drink this water, once it goes in, I have the feeling that not only it is cleaning up my contaminated guts but also it is cleaning up my dirty mind. I hope all the readers of this book have this experience, drinking the best of the good. You will have a once-in-a-lifetime experience that you will never forget.

What is good water? We can safely say a well-cleaned, uncontaminated water would be good enough. It would be better if the water is boiled and cooled, supposedly bacteria free or germ free. Not too cold, not too hot. I recommend highly the kind of drinks like green tea which is proven to contain a high amount of antioxidant.

Then what is bad water? The worst example is those water that is "contaminated" with alcohol, also called whiskey, beer, and so on. If you drink this kind of water wisely, it can be good for your body.

But if you drink this "bad" water unwisely, it will be bad for your body and mind as well for sure. It will ruin your body and mind if you drink alcohol unwisely. We all know that. If we drink this bad water wisely, it will turn into good water for our body and mind. I do not have to explain any further because we all know very well already. Also, the bad ones are the water with caffeine, such as coffee and caffeinated soda, etc. Recently, it concerns me a lot that we see in commercials more and more the water called energy drink. It is being called "energy," but what energy is it providing to our young people who think it is cool to drink this false energy?

In recent studies, researchers report that too hot water may be harmful to our body, although more studies need to be done. In my opinion, too cold water may not be good to our body either, more specifically to our stomach. I do not recommend people drinking soda, such as cola with ice, as often seen in commercials. If you want or have to drink cola with ice, drink it extremely slow. Likewise, in the hot summer sun, I do not encourage people drinking ice-cold beer, with a big smile as in beer commercials. You may feel good today, but certainly, your stomach will complain to you later on.

What is thirst? Why do we feel thirsty? When we feel thirsty, it comes with a subtle physical change at the same time. It is not just a feeling. Our mouth as well as tongue and lips get dry. Of course, our skin gets dry too. When we have certain conditions, we will end up having a serious illness related with water. Usually, water-related conditions come and go very quick. If you do not treat the patient immediately or in time, you can lose your patient real easy.

We can think of two conditions. One is that we have too much water in our body, and the other is the opposite—too little water. When we are talking about water in our body, we have to keep in mind electrolytes at the same time. So in the textbook, we call this condition fluid and electrolyte imbalance.

In a condition called fluid overload, it is either we drink too much or we do not eliminate fluid in time. Most of the time, with kidney disease or heart disease, we end up with a serious problem of fluid overload, like chronic renal failure or congestive heart failure.

And now the other extreme is fluid depleted or dehydrated. It is when we have a condition that we eliminate fluid or water too much. And then we go into a condition called dehydration, which is one of fluid and electrolyte imbalance. In case of dehydration, based on severity, we classify this condition into three, which is mild, moderate, and severe.

In a case of severe dehydration, people can die, particularly in pediatric population. Even with simple diarrhea alone, newborn babies die easily. This condition is a pediatric emergency and a pediatrician's nightmare.

Here, what we are going to discuss about is a mild case of dehydration as a result of not drinking enough water, with which we are not dealing with a life-or-death situation. But it can be serious and potentially dangerous with the geriatric population.

Unfortunately, our body does not have an early warning system of any dehydration. Instead, we have a late warning system, which means by the time we get the warning signal, i.e., thirst, it is already too late. By the time, our cells cry out loud that they are thirsty and dehydrated and the desperate message goes to our brain, tongue, and lips, our cells are already on the verge of death, somewhere in between life and death. Some of our cells are no longer alive because of dehydration. And yet most of us ignore even this late warning signal of thirst. So to prevent this preventable, unnecessary tragedy from happening, we have to drink a small amount of water as frequently as possible.

I grew up in a culture where the seniors, mostly parents, encourage not to drink water. They discourage water drinking especially in the evening or before going to bed. Most likely, the reason for this culture might have originated from preventing bed-wetting at night. Always my parents made sure to tell me, "Don't drink before you go to bed!" Yes, you need to drink, otherwise. To drink wisely is important. Then you need to go to the bathroom before you go to bed.

When we are having a serious meeting, either business or religious, it does not look good if somebody disrupts the flow of the meeting to go to the bathroom.

Earlier, I emphasized that our body has twice as much water than the solid portion. So I can hardly emphasize more about the enormous importance of water in our body. Everything goes into our body mixed with water or water alone and comes out mixed with water, such as sweat, urine, and stool. In a way, our body is like a water balloon with perhaps some dust inside.

So again, I have to say we have to drink a little and as frequent as possible. I do not know how little is little and how frequent is frequent. These are all subjective. Your little can be too much for me. Somebody's too much can be too little for me. Your frequent can be not frequent for me. My frequent can be not frequent for somebody. This has to be individualized. You have to come up with your own little amount of water and frequency. I have to come up with my little amount of water and frequency. Because we cannot see inside our cells to tell how much and when the cells are in need of water.

It is not good and I do not recommend drinking a large amount of water at a time. Whatever the reason is, when we are thirsty, i.e., dehydrated, we drink a lot. In this situation, I would still recommend to drink a little and more frequently. Why? If we drink a large amount of water at a time, exactly like a balloon, our stomach has to expand, so the wall of our stomach has to stretch. This is when our stomach pumps out the digestive enzymes and gastric acid. In this situation, our stomach has no defense from the acid and enzymes. We have nothing to neutralize the acid that our own stomach produced. The gastric acid will hurt your stomach wall real bad and destroy the barrier, and the enzymes will digest our own cells. When and if you eat, the food you ate will act as antacid. The food itself will act as antacid that neutralizes the acid. So it is more dangerous to have gastric acid pouring out after drinking a lot of water at a time than after eating a big meal because the food is neutralizing the acid to some extent. In general, this is the reason why beer drinkers are having more stomach problem and/or pancreatic problem than whiskey drinkers, who generally are having more liver problem.

I do agree that little bit of alcohol is good for our body and mind, but I rarely see many of us have the ability to control the amount of alcohol once we start drinking. When we drink alcohol, we often see three groups of people. The first group are people drinking alcohol. People enjoy alcohol. People control alcohol. Most of us belong to this group. And next is the second group, which is alcohol drinking alcohol. Alcohol controls people. Then the third group is alcohol drinking people. Alcohol controls humans. But both humans and alcohol go out of control, and no one knows who is in charge. The alcohol says, "I'm in charge and in control, human."

I do not understand why people are competing how much they can drink. Even though I was born with no or a little alcoholic gene that I rarely drink alcohol more than I want, I have no problem with people drinking alcohol to get high as much as they want. But I have a big problem with those people who drink more than as much as they want called alcoholic, which is being controlled by alcohol. Why do you have to be called alcoholic? As I said, I have no problem with people drinking alcohol as much as to get high, i.e., to feel good or feel better. I do have a big problem with people who have to drink more than as much as they need, either to show off their manhood, such as in college campuses, or to express their anger or for no reason whatsoever at all. If someone needs the help of alcohol other than the reason to get high, i.e., to feel good, they need the help of psychiatrists, psychologists, priests, or ministers, not alcohol.

It's about time to conclude. We are made of and made from water. And when we were being made, we were in the water also. Then after a while when the time for us to go back comes, we all go back to water. Only one-third of us go back to the dust.

So when and if we lose a certain amount of water, we can get sick easily, and/or we can die easily. Just look at a newborn baby; they can die real easy with a simple diarrhea only, which is the worst nightmare of pediatricians and/or pediatric residents. For the grownups, we think we have an early warning signal also known as thirst, which is very unreliable that by the time we feel thirsty, it could be already too late at cellular level. In an ordinary situation, when we have drinking water around us, we rarely die because of dehydration itself. But in the worst scenario, we can die due to dehydration when the water intake stops and/or too much water is lost.

In this chapter, we are discussing water in an ordinary setting. We are not going to die just because we are thirsty. We are trying to make a good water turn into the best water for me and for all of us, which is to drink wisely. Drink *a little and as frequently* as possible!

CHAPTER 6

Tutankhamen, Also Known as King Tut

When you visit Cairo, the capital city of Egypt, you will go to the Museum of Egyptian Antiquities, also known as Museum of Cairo, one of the must-see tourist attractions in Egypt.

At the entrance of the museum, you have to give up all your photographic equipment, including iPhone, and then receive a ticket to retrieve your belongings when you leave. There are many places where you are not allowed to take photos, but this one is the only rare place that you have to turn in your photo equipment.

Once you get in, it is not allowed for anyone to talk loud inside, especially for the tour guides to speak loud to their group. So our tour guide told us to sit down on the stairs of the first floor and explained about what to see, what we should not miss, and so on. Then we were set free. We were on our own to look around. We were feeling a bit upset or annoyed because we could not take any pictures at all, and we could not talk to each other either, in case our voice would go high.

My freedom of speech and my freedom of recording were well restricted and taken away. I do not understand why so many places are restricting photos. What kind of damage does it give to paintings, sculptures, antiques, and so on by taking pictures without flashes? Or even with flashes. Some scientists have to do a research about what is the potential damage about being the object of photos. If taking pictures can cause damage to a lifeless object, what about us? We are living humans. I never heard of any movie stars who died at the end of their career because they were exposed to too much taking pictures.

Anyway, while listening to the guide, most of us, especially the very sensitive-minded people of our group, could not help but have a few tears in our eyes.

After the tour guide—who made us sure to see the flowers on the top of the sarcophagus of King Tut that was given by his wife, the queen—finished her speeches, we were all free to go around wherever we wanted to go in the four-story building. It is quite a big building. If two or three of the four floors are filled with and came from one person's burial site or tomb, who is going to believe that? This is an excellent example of how powerful and how rich a pharaoh can be. A pharaoh had absolute political power, military leadership, and religious authority and was at the same level with God, and he owned everything in the country. This is why the name is Pharaoh Tutankhamun (or Tutankhamen)—meaning, "living image of Amun," the sun god.

So the pharaoh had three absolute powers in one individual—political, military, and religious.

First, like any other leader, he is on the top of everyone in the country. He is the country. Sometimes he designates this power to someone else, such as his son or loyal follower, to focus on the more important issues as he is also the religious leader. Even so, he still holds the ultimate power.

Second, simultaneously, he is the military leader. He is the commander in chief. The difference is when there is a war, he does not stay behind. He himself goes to war, not his son or his general. Even at war, he always stays in the front, not behind. Even if the pharaoh dies in the battlefield, they never say, "Pharaoh died while fighting the enemy" because a pharaoh does not die. God never dies. You cannot find in any records documenting that a pharaoh died as a result of a disease, war, or old age, etc., because he is God, not a human being. God does not die. Another difference compared to other countries is that Egypt, i.e., the pharaoh, had a standing military force ready to go to war all the time. Not like the rest of the other countries or the rest of the world that only have generals and a few elite forces during a peaceful period that when there is a war, ordinary people become the main force voluntarily or involuntarily. Egypt was opposite. It had a standing army ready to go to war any time and all the time. Always ready to go to war. Generals and soldiers, the war professionals, are always ready to kill enemies. Financially, it could afford to have, keep, and maintain a huge standing army that is physically and mentally ready to kill the enemies. They are killing machines. The Roman Empire had the same military system as with the Egyptian Army.

Third, as mentioned above, he is God. The pharaoh is not human. No further explanation is necessary to find out what kind of power he has. He is the one and only highest priest as well who does not die.

Fourth, the Egyptians were rich, which means the pharaoh, who owned the country, was rich. The river Nile gave the Egyptians more than enough wealth to become the strongest country in that part of the world. Two rivers from the south—one is from Ethiopia, and another one is from Kilimanjaro—become the long Nile river, which overflows twice a year and brings to Egypt nutritious, rich soil. They have plenty of harvests of grains twice a year. That's why Egypt could afford to have a standing army, always ready to fight and kill the enemies. They made their living by fighting and killing the enemies.

So when famine spread to the Middle East and even to Eastern Europe, people came to Egypt to get food or moved and stayed in Egypt until the crisis was over. To the people of the Middle East or Eastern Europe, Egypt was filled with peace and abundant foods.

Even for political reasons, Jesus came down to Cairo with his parents and lived from a few to many years in Egypt. We do not know exactly how long the holy family stayed and lived in Egypt.

Not to mention that there was a threat from other countries even in peaceful periods, the pharaoh took his army and went to war twice a year, once to the north, such as countries in the Middle East.

The most frequent target was Lebanon. And once to the south, such as Ethiopia and Sudan and so on.

We cannot compare the civilization of the Egyptian culture with any other cultures in the history of humanity because the Egyptians from the beginning had their own alphabets, language, unique art, military system, not to mention medicine, geometry, agriculture, etc., that other cultures did not have.

The civilization of the Mesopotamian culture is almost a thousand years longer than the Egyptian culture, but their culture has almost nothing or little left behind. Egypt had to be far superior to any other cultures in terms of national wealth, military strength, religious authority, etc. The Egyptian culture has almost everything left because the culture is written on the stone, and everything are mummified due to the desert weather.

When the Roman Empire became strong and powerful, the Romans learned and copied everything from the Greeks. The Greeks learned and copied everything from the Egyptians. In Rome, you cannot be a scholar, general, politician, scientist, etc., if you did not go to Greece and learn or if you did not have a teacher from Greece and learn. When the Greeks became strong and powerful, they learned and copied from the Egyptians. Exactly what the Romans did from the Greeks, the Greeks did exactly the same from the Egyptians.

Geographically, Egypt is well protected from outside enemies. Occasionally being invaded from the north and the south is the reason why the pharaoh would bring his army to the north once and to the south once annually to show off the strength of the Egyptian military.

In the east, there is the Red Sea, then Saudi Arabia. Saudi Arabia is a country of desert with no kingdom or solid national system. Even if it does, it does not have big trees to make good ships. So Saudis do not have a strong navy. If one has no big trees, one has no good ship and no strong navy.

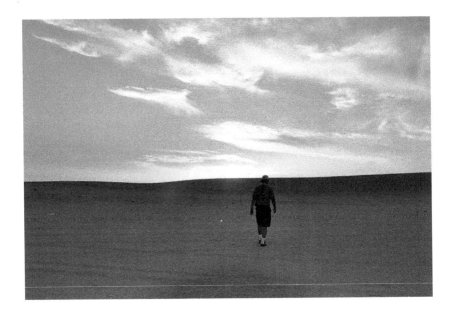

In the west, there is the Sahara desert protecting Egypt. The desert that is practically impossible to cross is protecting Egypt. Egyptians never crossed the desert. No enemy ever crossed the desert. Even if they were to cross the desert, they would have no strength left to fight the strong enemy. They would be lucky if they could go back home. They would have to cross the same desert.

From the north, occasionally, Egypt was invaded. They put the Egyptian military on the northern border, and furthermore once a year, the pharaoh would bring his army to the north and made sure they could not even think about invading Egypt. So throughout the history of Egypt up until the era of Cleopatra, Egypt did not have any serious threat from the north, not to mention from the south, east, or west.

To the south, such as Sudan or Ethiopia, the pharaoh of course would bring his army annually. But the problem is defending the border. Of course, the best defense is offense. That's what they did every year. But it was practically impossible to go to war all the time. And the southern border of Egypt is too wide and too long to station militaries to protect it.

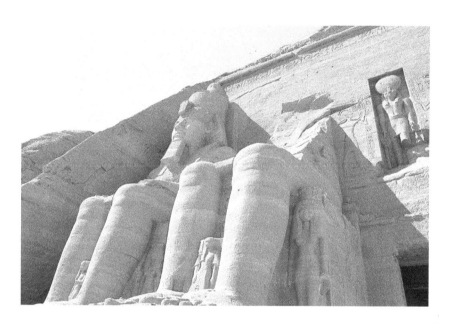

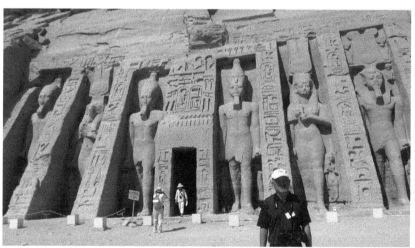

So in addition to the annual offense, Ramses the Great constructed Abu Simbel on the top of a rocky mountain at the southern border. He built gigantic statues of himself and the sun god outside and inside the cave. And next to his temple, he built another temple dedicated to his wife, the queen. So he constructed two gigantic temples with huge statues at the very strategic spot where the enemies coming from the south had to pass the Abu Simbel, a symbol of power.

If you stand in front of this structure, the temple on the mountain, immediately you will feel that they are big and huge and you are small and tiny. You cannot help but feel you are so tiny, and they, the Egyptians, are huge and gigantic. As a result, if you are the enemy of Egypt and you are the leader of the invading force, immediately you are going to lose the fighting will, which will disappear at once like an ice in a hot summer sun. And you will get homesick right away. You will want to see your family before your certain death. Immediately, you will want to see your family back home. You will think about not being able to see your family left behind. You will want to go home after dropping your weapons to the ground and turn around. But as a tourist or as a visitor, no sooner you stand in front of the gigantic structure than you cannot help but feel your heart and your mind become empty and get humbled by the great achievement of our fellow human beings, although we were born in a different time and different place.

Even though I visited many different places and saw many structures, small and huge, when I stood in front the Abu Simbel, my jaw dropped to the ground, and I could not find it even though I wanted to shut my mouth.

Twice a year, on a particular day in the spring and in the fall, when the sun rises, the ray of sunshine comes into the cave and drops at the right shoulder of Ramses the Great. According to the tour guide, on those two days, myriad of tourists come to Abu Simbel the day or two days before, many of them camping on the ground in front of the entrance and waiting for the time.

In fact, the art of stone carving originated from Egypt, then spread to the Greeks who learned from the Egyptians. Then the

Greeks spread the art to the Romans and to the rest of Europe and the world. Especially Alexander the Great was the one who spread this stone art form from Europe to India. Then from India to China. From China to Korea. And finally, from Korea to Japan. I still remember that we used to buy a seal, like a postage stamp, from school when I was in elementary school.

It was an effort to save Abu Simbel from drowning, i.e., going underwater, when the Egyptian government of Gamal Abdel Nasser was building the Aswan Dam in the area of Abu Simbel. The UNESCO (United Nations Educational, Scientific and Cultural Organization) was the one that organized the movement to save Abu Simbel. They meticulously cut the mountain rock one meter by one meter by one meter and moved it to above the water level where they are now.

As a matter of fact, modern-time Egyptians are not Egyptians. They are Arabs. Actually, the real Egyptians are from down south of Africa, who followed up the water route of Nile river. Strictly speaking, Egyptians are Africans, and majority of the Egyptians in Egypt now are Arabs. So in the present time of Egypt, most of the so-called Egyptians are Arabs who came down from the Middle East or farther north from countries like Iran or Saudi Arabia.

In modern history, when someone becomes the president of Egypt, even though they do not know for sure whether they are a true Egyptian or not, they feel like or act like a pharaoh. What an irony we are looking at.

But in the history of Egypt, many of the heroes in Europe or the Mediterranean region desperately wanted to become the pharaoh of Egypt. Anyone who becomes a strong man wants to be the ruler of Egypt, the pharaoh.

First of all, we can pick Alexander the Great of Macedonia. His father, the king of Macedon, was assassinated when he was twenty years old or less, and he then took over the throne. He continued his father's battle and defeated the mighty Persians, whose leader was the great king Darius III (333 BC). Then he went to Egypt as a liberator, not as a conqueror, and became an Egyptian to be the pharaoh of Egypt. As a field general, he never lost a single battle until he died at the age of thirty when he was coming back from India. Egypt was then given to one of his trusted generals, Ptolemy. So for the next three hundred years or so, until the fall of the Egyptian Empire, Egypt was ruled by the Greeks, not by the Egyptians.

And next is my favorite person in the history of the Roman Empire, Julius Caesar, who became a pharaoh by marrying another pharaoh and also the inventor of the Nile river cruise with Cleopatra, which we are copying two thousand years later. He was born in July in 100 BC and was assassinated by his fellow men in March in 44 BC, who were afraid that Caesar was becoming too powerful as one person. He transformed single-handedly the Roman Republic to the Roman Empire, where one individual held all the power as emperor instead of the senate where many individuals shared the power. As a military leader, he conquered and expanded the territory to the modern-day France and Belgium and made Rome even bigger than before, even stronger than before, and, more importantly, even safer than before. As a political leader, with the help of the ever-rising popularity of all the Romans, he started eliminating his political opponents and concentrating the power on one person, himself.

Pompeius, the leader of the republicans and the head of the main opposition of Caesar, fled to Egypt. Caesar followed him. But Pompeius was already assassinated by Cleopatra's brother, for fear that he might be blamed if Pompeius was still alive. Then he himself was killed by Caesar. By then, the entire world knew who had the ultimate power.

Two MIPs (most important persons or most influential persons) in the history of humanity—of course, one is Jesus Christ, and the other is Julius Caesar—who impacted immensely on people's lives then and even now might have met each other in Egypt if Jesus was born a bit sooner.

Now the superpower of the world moved to the Roman Empire, not Egypt. The superpower of the Roman Empire was concentrated on one person, Julius Caesar. By the time Caesar came to Egypt, he already became the most powerful man of the world. In Egypt, there was a power struggle between the siblings, but the one who got the attention and support of Caesar became the winner of the power struggle.

Cleopatra—young, talented, intelligent, and beautiful—became the pharaoh of Egypt after eliminating her sister and brother with the help of Caesar.

In Rome, all the citizens were anxiously waiting for the triumphant return of their hero. But there was no sign of their hero's return. Instead, all they were hearing was that their hero got married to the Egyptian queen and consequently became God. And they, the two gods, were honeymooning on the Nile river in the first Nile river cruise or any cruise in the world history.

It was a political marriage for Cleopatra, who needed a powerful figure behind her to govern her country. She was in her early twenties, and Caesar was in his fifties. We all know who was controlling who. We all know who was in charge.

The Romans knew better and better and more and more than anybody else, and they were getting angry. But instead of hating or getting angry at Caesar, the Romans chose to hate Cleopatra. They began to destroy any statues or paintings of Cleopatra if there was any. That is the reason why we do not see any of her face or entire body painting or statues.

By the time their hero returned to Rome with Cleopatra, he became or was already not only the emperor of the Roman Empire in reality but also the pharaoh of Egypt. So to the eyes of the patriotic Romans, Julius Caesar was not one of their own anymore. He had too much power and wanted to be God and was already God. To the ordinary Romans, he was too dangerous and going out of control. And they did something that they regretted right away. The ordinary people killed their own god. Immediately, they knew what they did was something bad, really bad. "And you know the rest of the story. Have a good day."

Third, the one who tried to be a pharaoh but failed. This individual is a French hero, whose name is Napoleon Bonaparte, who was born in 1769 and died in 1821. After a triumphant return from Italy, he planned to invade England, which was his longtime dream and also for all the people of France. As his plan got more practical, he realized it was practically next to impossible to achieve because he did not have decent naval forces to cross over the channel or the Strait of Dover and invade England or engage in a naval warfare with the British if necessary. He did not know much about war at sea. And the other reason is he was an artillery officer.

So instead, he decided to invade Egypt to block the Suez Canal so that the merchant ships or military vessels of England had to sail around the African continent to go to India and come back to the same route. His strategy was to give a significant blow to the economy of England and wait until the appropriate time to attack.

But this was not the only reason that he wanted to occupy Egypt. He wanted to do exactly what his personal heroes, Alexander the Great and Julius Caesar, did—to be the pharaoh of Egypt. At that time, he was only twenty-nine years old. He was a very ambitious man as we all know, and nothing's going to stop him.

He came to Egypt not only with his military force but also with a bunch of nonmilitary personnel for the exact purpose unknown. He brought approximately 150 scientists with him. Of course, many were archeologists, and some were artists.

He went to Egypt, forced out the Turkish military who was defending Egypt, and occupied Egypt briefly. It was only brief because Admiral Nelson came to the rescue of Egypt from French occupation because he knew better than anybody else the importance of Suez Canal militarily and economically. He wasted no time.

But as soon as Napoleon's army occupied Egypt, they began a huge excavation, collecting as many antiques as possible. Soon, there was Admiral Nelson, a naval warfare genius, who recognized the seriousness of the blockade of the Suez Canal. He, Admiral Nelson himself, showed up with his fleet. And as a result, Napoleon's entire fleet sank to the bottom of the sea, which was later called the Battle of the Nile.

Napoleon had to escape to Paris without achieving the biggest dream of his life, i.e., becoming the pharaoh of Egypt. Although his mission ended up in total failure, with the help of an extremely poor communication and a total lack of mass media, he received a hero's welcome in Paris because he told the country that he liberated Egypt with great military success. Then to distract the people's attention away from his failure in Egypt, he invaded Russia, which happened to be the beginning of his downfall and demise.

By the way, about the time he was receiving a hero's welcome and marching through the streets of Paris, the rest of the troops and the scientists who were captured and became prisoners of war by Nelson were receiving as much humiliation as Napoleon's hero's welcome. They were ordered to give up and turn in to Nelson every antique that they had excavated and collected.

At the negotiation table, the commanding general representing the French Army had no choice but to turn in everything they had. He made an offer or a request to Nelson to give everything except the Rosetta Stone that they found, but Nelson was firm. Nelson was so firm that they were very lucky that they returned to Paris without losing their lives. Every item that they collected, including the Rosetta Stone, was given to Nelson and brought to London rather than to Paris. And you know the rest of the story. We all know that who the owner of the Rosetta stone is and in what museum it is kept since then.

The history of Egypt, as we know, began in 3100 BC when Pharaoh Narmer united the north and south of Egypt. So Narmer built the Old Kingdom, which lasted for about one thousand years. Then came the first Intermediate Period (2181 to 2049 BC), and then came the Middle Kingdom (2134 to 1782 BC). Then came the Second Intermediate Period (1782 to 1650 BC), and the latest came the New Kingdom.

At the end of the New Kingdom, in 332 BC, Egypt was conquered by Alexander the Great and was ruled by the Greeks until 30 BC when Cleopatra who is a Greek, the last pharaoh of Egypt, was married to Julius Caesar, who became the first emperor of the Roman Empire and also the last pharaoh of Egypt.

Officially, the history of Egypt ended in 32 BC, but practically, it ended way three hundred years earlier in 332 BC.

At the peak of the New Kingdom, there was a pharaoh whose name was Amenhotep IV. Later, he changed his name to Akhenaten (and ruled Egypt from 1350 to 1334 BC), which means "effective for Aten." He is the father of King Tut, who is the main character of this chapter. Unlike the tradition, he was married to a commoner, Nefertiti, who was the most beautiful woman in the history of Egypt. Based on the record, some archeologists claim she is more beautiful than Cleopatra, which makes her the most beautiful woman who ever lived in this planet in the history of mankind. When he changed his name, he began to preach there is only one god, Aten.

Typically, Egypt had been a country of multiple gods and a very progressive and open-minded society. All of a sudden, the people of Egypt were told by their living god that there is only one god, Aten. But there was no bloody conflict between one god, Aten, and the rest of the gods. They maintained a peaceful coexistence, which happens to be entirely different from what is happening in the present world of the twenty-first century.

Those who believe and claim that there is only one god and nothing else must go back to the history of Egypt and learn from Akhenaten, the most generous, open-minded, and one and only religious leader in the entire human history who allowed the existence of other gods or other religions from the beginning till the present day of humanity. It is amazing to see the difference and remarkably shameful reality between what he had done as god over more than three thousand years ago and what is being done now or what we are doing in the modern days of the twenty-first century. There was no political, social, or religious turmoil between the two—monotheism versus polytheism. Not even a single life had been lost simply because they, the rest of Egyptians, worshipped other gods or different gods. He had all the power and authority to suppress and wipe out other religions but chose not to. He accepted the existence of other gods. It appears that the god and pharaoh allowed his people to worship other gods other than Aten, his one and only god. God, the pharaoh, allowed his people the freedom to worship other gods. This is absolutely unacceptable in any religion, or at least between two religions in the twenty-first century.

Then he built a new holy city and capital two hundred miles away from Thebes in the middle of the Sahara Desert, Tell el-Amarna. He moved from the capital city with his followers from Thebes to the new city that he built with his followers, those who believed in Aten like he did.

This is a revolution, the one and only true revolution. No one was put into jail, and no one died, not even one single soul. No one shed a single drop of blood. Indeed, archeologists call this entire event Amarna revolution. There are many revolutions in the history of the world, but there is no revolution as radical as this one, and yet no one died. Again, this single event shows exactly how powerful a pharaoh is. But modern-day so-called religious leaders must learn from him on how to coexist with other religions even while believing in the one and only god of their own.

He had three daughters with Nefertiti, the most beautiful woman in the history of Egypt or, as I claimed, in the history of mankind. If she is more beautiful than Cleopatra, there is no one beyond her.

He had a son, Tutankhamen, in his later life with his minor wife, Kiya. Unfortunately, Akhenaten died when King Tut was only eight years old. Tutankhamen became the pharaoh of Egypt at the young age of eight and then married his two years' older half sister, Ankhesenamun. According to the tradition of Egypt, in order to be a legitimate pharaoh, you have to marry the first daughter of the pharaoh. This is the most legitimate way to become a pharaoh.

Although a marriage within the royal family does have an advantage, it simultaneously has invisible disadvantages. If you marry within the royal family, the power remains within the family. But if you marry within the family, it has a high probability for genetic mutations or genetic defects. As a result, there is a high incidence of stillbirth, genetic disease, and hereditary disease.

By the way, what did he know about religion or politics or anything as an eight-year-old boy? And what did his young queen know about religion or politics as a ten-year-old girl?

At the time, Egypt had pharaohs, the king and the queen, but the country was ruled by the king's adviser, the prime minister, Ay, who moved the capital back to Thebes.

The young couple grew up together like siblings. Practically, they are half brother and half sister with the same father. Apparently, they had two babies, but they appeared to be stillborn. Then Tutankhamen died suddenly when he was eighteen years only. For the cause of his death, there are two theories: one is due to infection, gangrene of his leg, and the other is murder. He was killed by someone. By who?

First, he died of some kind of infectious disease untreatable with ancient medicine that they had to watch him die slowly. The most likely cause of his death was a massive gangrene of the lower extremities due to wound infection inflicted in a fight with enemies or during strenuous physical activities. The scientists who investigated the cause of his death now agreed that there was no evidence of skull fracture or hematoma inside his skull based on X-rays and CAT scans.

Second, King Tut was too young to govern Egypt, the superpower of northern Africa and the Middle East. Quite naturally, the pharaoh's adviser, the prime minister Ay, was the one who controlled everything. He was the ruler of Egypt behind the young pharaoh. As King Tut grew older, it is just a matter of time that Ay had to give up all the power he had back to the fast-growing young pharaoh. So the pharaoh's fate was at the hands of his "best" man. He planned to kill the pharaoh, then forced the queen to marry him. Then he announced to the nation that he himself was the legitimate pharaoh, so then no one would object the god.

Of course, the country would never believe the pharaoh was dead or killed by someone. They would believe the young pharaoh went to the next world to have a more meaningful life. In the history of any country, when the king or emperor was betrayed by his best man, the king was the most vulnerable. So as he planned, Ay committed the perfect crime and buried the young pharaoh in a hurry. Usually, a pharaoh's funeral would last at least a few years. But King Tut's funeral must have lasted for a few months only or much less than that. The tomb he was buried was already made for someone else and available at the time he died.

During the funeral, the queen went to the Nile river and picked up beautiful flowers with her own hands. She laid the flowers on the top of King Tut's sarcophagus. When King Tut's tomb was found untouched in 1922 by Howard Carter, people found the mummified flowers on the top of King Tut's sarcophagus. When King Tut's body was mummified, the flowers were also mummified with him. Most likely, the grieving heart of the young queen became mummified with her husband's body. When tourists see these mummified flowers, people become a bit emotional, including myself.

Now the young queen had to marry the old prime minister and was very afraid of him. Because she knew who murdered her husband and why. Just imagine how scary it would be for the young woman, about twenty years old, to be living with someone who killed her young husband. And the person, who was more than sixty years old and murderer of her husband, wanted to marry her? How did the archeologists find out about this plot? There is evidence, not direct but indirect. She sent a letter to the king of the Hittites, saying she was willing to be married to one of his sons, which the king agreed. He accepted the offer that one of his sons would be the next pharaoh of Egypt and sent one to Egypt to marry the queen.

But the prince never showed up in Egypt. The prince and his soldiers were ambushed and murdered while at sleep by a group of small and strong army in civilian clothes in the middle of the night just before they were to cross the border. The king of Hittites could not blame or protest formally to Egypt because the prince and his army were killed outside of Egypt's border by an unknown group of "assassins," and there were no witnesses left behind. But the archeologists know that the prince was sent to Egypt because this event was written in the history of the country of Hittites.

Unfortunately, King Tut died young. The queen died also soon after the "best loyal person" of her husband became the next pharaoh when her name disappeared from the record. That means the person is not existing any longer.

But King Tut got lucky after he died. Because no one touched his burial site and his tomb. There is not even a single pharaoh's tomb untouched, except King Tut's. There are so many pharaohs in the history of Egypt and so many pharaohs' tombs. But no pharaoh's tomb is untouched, except this one.

The very explanation for the reason that we, i.e., archeologists, can think of—as some archeologists speculate—is when a pharaoh's tomb was built and completed, before long the very people who built the tomb who knew what's in the tomb came back and took away the valuables. And then when the people's interest or curiosity was enhanced by the discovery of the Rosetta Stone, the excavation and collection of Egyptian antiques became a hot commodity and much more rampant than ever.

Ever since the fall of Cleopatra, Egypt was owned by the Roman Empire, more specifically by the emperor of Rome, then by the Muslims from Arab countries, which means Egypt was a country but without a government of its own. So any countries or any persons who come to Egypt and collect the antiques automatically and quite naturally become the owner of whatever they collected.

Anyway, if you visit national Museum of Cairo without the knowledge of King Tut, even after you spent your hard-earned money and time, when you went inside the museum and came out, you would be the same person before and after. No improvement. But if you visit the museum with the knowledge of King Tut, by the time you come out of the building, you will be a different person, at least emotionally. Anytime you are thinking of your valuable trip to Egypt and this young couple whose love story was abruptly cut short, at least you can pray for them to your god that they continue their love story for a long, long time together in their next life.

CHAPTER 7

Pepcid

Wake up in the morning and take one baby aspirin. And before you go to bed, take one Pepcid. Start your day with aspirin and finish your day with Pepcid.

I'm going to explain the reason why we should take aspirin in the chapter "Aspirin." But in this chapter, I'll explain why we should take one Pepcid at night.

The reason why I advocate about Pepcid is to protect our poor stomach, the most abused organ in our body. Unlike other organs, the stomach is abused the most inhumanely but never complains to the owner. Since we cannot witness the moment of abuse and barely feel the consequences of abuse until we face the real tragedy of our abuse, the abuse will continue and will never stop. We are in a big trouble when and if our loyal servant tells us, "I cannot or will not go on this way any longer."

We humans are the only animals who eat three times a day, sometimes more than three times a day, whether it rains or snows. Also, we humans are the only animals who eat not only for survival of our species but also for this pleasure of food taste itself. It is same in the issue of sexual activity, not only for the survival of our species but also for the pleasure itself. Humans are the only animals who do this activity for the pleasure itself. Alleluia!

And yet only humans cook foods with fire before eating and put all different ingredients together to make the food taste better.

So depending on the culture, we put so many different ingredients to the food. Thus, even if we use the same vegetables and meat, the taste would be entirely different with different ethnic cuisines.

Since I was born and raised in Korea, I have no other choice but to talk about Korean foods. I'm going to be honest when I talk about Korean foods. Generally speaking, Korean foods are one of the healthiest foods of all, if not the healthiest. So seeing is believing. Just go to a Korean restaurant and take a look at and taste the food. You will agree with me instantaneously. It's the best. The most popular dishes are bibimbap, *galbi* (grilled ribs), and bulgogi. Generally, the main dishes are a very high quality of cooked rice along with well-boiled soup, which is sometimes a many-hours boiled soup from bone and meat. And then you will see many and different brilliant side dishes, from which you will absorb all different kinds of nutrients. I'm talking about all the vitamins and minerals. Count the number of side dishes and compare it with that of any other restaurants, including Chinese, Japanese, Vietnamese, etc. Tell me if there is any ethnic restaurant that serves more side dishes than Korean restaurants. Simply, among Oriental restaurants, Chinese or Japanese included, how many side dishes do you see? Maybe none or one at most.

When you go to a Korean restaurant, if the waitress or waiter brings out one or two side dishes only, then you should immediately stand up and leave that place. But it will never happen, to be honest with you, because you will see four or more at any Korean restaurant you go. And if you like any of the side dishes, if and when you finish one side dish or more, ask your waitress or waiter to give you more. The servers are more than happy to give you more. There is no extra charge for additional side dishes. Do not hesitate to ask for more side dishes if you like. Sometimes, even before you ask for more, if the waitress recognizes your side dish is empty, she will ask you if you want to have more of that particular side dish. That is the core of Korean culture—that something you like will be given to you before you ask for it, with no additional charge. You do not need to say anything. Just make an eye contact with the waitress and point your finger to the empty dishes. If they charge you for the side dishes, just give me a call. That's all you have to do to receive additional side dishes—make eye contact and point with your handsome finger. That's all you need.

So far, I mentioned the good side of Korean food and culture. Although it is impossible to list all the good aspects of Korean food and culture, I have done my best.

Now let's talk about the negative aspects of Korean food and culture. This is how Koreans are assaulting their own stomachs. There are three ways of assaulting our stomach in general—first, the way the food is prepared; second, the quantity of one meal; and third and last but not the least, the speed.

First, let's talk about the way the food is prepared. The food is spicy and salty. This is the main character of Korean food. The saltier and the spicier, the better the taste will be. I do not mean to say that all Korean foods are spicy and salty and that only Korean foods are salty and spicy. There are many other Korean dishes which are not salty or spicy at all. And of course, there are many other ethnic foods which are much saltier and spicier than Korean food.

In terms of spicy food, a friend of mine from India gave me a treat with a very high quality of curry. Yes, indeed, it was so spicy that it burned and then numbed my tongue and lips for hours, probably my entire gastrointestinal tract also. It was may be one of the spiciest foods I ever had in my life. I can definitely and respectably say that the spiciness of Korean food is no match for the spiciness of Indian food.

In terms of spiciness of food, I'd like to talk about the jalapeño of Turkey, the spiciest and hottest jalapeño of all, not the Mexican one we are familiar with. In my experience, the Korean jalapeño is no match against the Mexican jalapeño, and the Mexican jalapeño is no match against the Turkish jalapeño. Because I have never seen a person passing out, literally losing consciousness, while eating jalapeño except this one, the Turkish jalapeño.

I personally almost passed out while eating this Turkish hot pepper. One of my traveling companions literally passed out while eating this. It happened few years ago when I was traveling in Turkey in a group tour. One day, at the end of the day, we arrived at our hotel for dinner and much-needed rest and relaxations. It was one of the best hotels in the city, if not the best. There was even live music by traditional musicians to stimulate our appetites. The dinner was a buffet. It was wonderful. There was so much to enjoy—big piece of beef steak, fresh and crispy vegetables, and so on. The foods were fantastic. I picked up a few of the very good—and innocent-looking jalapeños. Unfortunately and fortunately, I started my dinner with jalapeño. At the moment I crushed the jalapeño and even before chewing, I felt a burning sensation in my mouth, which I've never felt before in my entire life. I thought it was one of the worst enemies of mine that sneaked on me from behind and threw a gasoline bomb into my mouth. Instantaneously, I became blind although my eyes were wide open, and my eyes were profusely watering. At the same time, I became deaf. I could not hear any sound, although I cleaned my ears in the shower that morning. I could not feel anything, although my nervous system was perfectly within normal range in my annual physical exam. My brain stopped functioning, and nothing was going on inside my brain. My mind went blank. I do not know how long the time passed.

As I recall, I was in a position that I looked like I was praying before a meal, as if I were a devoted Christian. When I realized what happened, I gave a desperate warning to the people in my table. And then the moment I was going to stand up to make a public announcement to the rest of the group not to eat any of the jalapeño if they picked up any of them, I was a bit too late. There was a sharp screaming coming from behind my table. It was from one of the ladies who might happen to be a soprano singer in her church choir. When I turned around, I saw a lady lying down comfortably on the floor with her arms and legs stretched, pointing to all four directions. Apparently, the lady took one bite out of the same kind of jalapeño I had and passed out. And the soprano scream was not from the lady on the floor; it was from another lady sitting next to her, the victim of the same jalapeño that I had a few minutes or a few seconds earlier. She was well attended by three well-experienced physicians, including myself, and two others in our tour group. As a result, the ambulance crew came and went empty-handed.

As I mentioned earlier, a Korean meal has more side dishes than any other ethnic meals, which can be salty and spicy also, like the way main meals are cooked. This can be good for the tongue but bad for the stomach simultaneously. For the best example for side dish, have you tried kimchi before? Some kimchis can be very hot and can be very salty. That is the reason why Korean foods are tastier and becoming ever more popular than any other country's foods—because they are hot and salty.

I have to mention several of the American and European foods also. People who like these foods are almost at an addiction level, not knowing how much salt there is in it or they are madly in love with salt. The first one is bacon. A lot of people like this food, including myself, and are almost addicted. Especially in the morning, if you are in a good hotel, you will be served with a well-cooked, crispy bacon, and you notice that people go crazy. I'm one of them. The other one is green olives. Olives itself are one of the healthiest foods of all. But I do not understand why it was made that salty. The green olives are very salty. On the other hand, the black olives are not salty, which are one of my favorite foods of all.

It is humans only who cook food with fire and put all different ingredients to make the food taste better. So the cooking became part of the culture among all the countries.

Geopolitically, Korea is located between China and Japan. Most likely, the Koreans took the advantage of both countries' cultures, particularly in food and cooking. Go to the kitchen and take a look at the cooking knife of each of these three countries. You can tell the difference immediately, and you will understand what I'm trying to say. The Japanese cooking knife is slim and razor-sharp. The Chinese cooking knife is the opposite. The Korean cooking knife is just in the middle. Just take a look and you will see how different the end product or food itself that comes out of these three different-looking cooking knives.

Additionally, to make the food tastier, Korean food contains lots of garlics. Probably among those countries, Korean cooking probably puts more garlics than any other countries in the world.

Of course, there are many other countries putting more garlics than Korean dishes.

This aspect again represents good and bad news to our body, specifically to our stomach.

Let us discuss the good news first. First, definitely, garlic makes the taste better. Yes, much better. It can give us the necessary natural defense against modern metabolic syndromes. Garlic is good for hypertension, diabetes, high cholesterol, etc. Garlic is also good against virus, especially against flu viruses. Garlic also gives us a good immune system. Even in flu epidemics all over Asian countries, the flu virus could not make any significant impact in the Korean Peninsula. The virus could not pass the "garlic checkpoint" in Incheon International Airport.

And these are the bad news. The garlic-rich Korean food or any garlic-rich food has bad news for the stomach. It is good for the tongue and mouth but bad for the stomach. This combination of the three musketeers—salt, hot pepper, and garlic—will make food tastier and increase the quality of human life to the limit but will make our stomach and the rest of our gastrointestinal tract pay the ultimate price. Statistics and the truth tell us that the incidence of gastrointestinal diseases in Korean population is one of the highest in the entire world. I do not mean to say we should not eat garlic-rich kimchi at all. But we have to protect our stomach at all costs, with the cost that does not cost us much or with a minimum cost. I am emphasizing that we have to consume those three elements—garlic, hot pepper, and salt—moderately but not excessively. If you eat too much of those three ingredients, you will end up facing a potential problem in the future for sure. We have to keep the truth in mind when we eat these. And take one Pepcid a day for our stomach.

Second, let's talk about the quantity, not quality, of the food we are eating in a meal at the table. The large amount of the food can give a big "headache" to our stomach. ADA (American Diabetes Association) advises people with diabetes to eat more frequently, which means smaller regular meals with snacks in between. This is exactly opposite of animals, especially meat-eating animals, i.e., carnivores.

When animals are not hungry, they do not eat. They eat only when they feel hungry. For example, the animals in the wilderness—such as tigers, lions, bears, and wolves, and so on—do not go out and hunt other animals for food when they are not hungry. They hunt only when and because they are hungry. Humans are the only animals that go out hunting for the pleasure of killing. We kill for the pleasure of killing itself. Animals go out hunting, i.e., killing, only because they are hungry. When tigers are not hungry, they do not hunt or kill, even when their best meal, i.e., wild rabbit, is playing right in front of their noses. We humans are the only creatures that kill other animals for the pleasure of killing itself.

Let's focus on the amount of meal we are eating. In general, among humans, we can divide two groups of people or cultures. There is one group of people or culture who mostly eat meats, a community that thrived in hunting animals in the past. And there is another group of people who mostly eat rice and vegetables, a community whose main means of providing food on the table is by means of agriculture.

If we compare these two cultures, the apparent difference between the two is the volume of each meal. In the meat-eating culture, you do not have to eat a lot of meat until your next meal or until you get hungry. It takes a long time to get hungry. But in the vegetables-and-rice-eating culture, you have to eat a large, literally huge, amount of vegetables but get hungry sooner or easier.

Now the trend of meals is moving toward more meat-eating pattern as the economy gets better. But up until a bit in the past, the typical Korean dinner consists of a bowl of rice—usually big and, at times, huge—soup, and four or more side dishes. So the ideal way of eating is to combine these two cultures together and meet somewhere in the middle. Imagine if you had a Big Mac with french fries and drink at lunch. Compared to a Korean meal or other vegetarian meal, a Big Mac meal takes a longer time to get you hungry until dinner. It also means you do not have to have a big meal in terms of volume.

The stomach does not have a brain. So it does not think. It only responds to certain stimuli. When the stomach is empty, it stays still or does not move. But something comes in from the above, and the wall of stomach is being stretched out. That's the time when it starts working. The stomach mixes the food slowly, then moves the food down to the next station. At the same time, our stomach is producing many digestive enzymes along with acid, a strong acid that can give first-degree, at times second-degree, burn to our skin. Literally, it can and will burn our skin. As a result of this, if the owner of the stomach happens to be a person who eats large or huge amount of meals, it is inevitable for the stomach to get stressed out and eventually end up with a significant and/or serious problem, which requires medical attention.

As I discussed before, simply because we do not see it with our own eyes, it takes long or longer sometimes. But if it's too late, no one knows when to recognize that there is some serious problem going on in our stomach.

We need to protect our poor stomach from all different kinds of assaults, like salty food, spicy food, food rich in garlic, food with pepper, and so on. I have a warning for those who love pepper. Remove the pepper bottle, which is the worst enemy of our stomach from the kitchen table. When I say "worst," it is worst.

We have to keep in mind that a large amount of meal can make our stomach work overtime. In the long run, there is much more potential to hurt the stomach than in smaller-meal culture.

It was a long, long time ago when the tigers were smoking pipes among humans. Actually, it was about fifty or so years ago when I was in senior year in medical school. It was a time when doctors had a real hard time treating peptic ulcer disease because there were not enough or almost no medicines to treat this disease. The situation was similar in the case of diabetes. There were no good diagnostic tools available at that time. But even if we make the correct diagnosis, there was little or almost no medicine available.

Now let us talk about peptic ulcer disease, then diabetes next.

Not only it was time that there was not enough or almost no medicine to treat but also there was not a single diagnostic tool to make accurate diagnosis, such as upper gastrointestinal endoscopy as currently available and used. So in those days, if somebody complained of upper abdominal pain or soreness, it was extremely difficult to differentiate peptic ulcer disease from other conditions causing similar kind of pain in similar location. Then in order to get some clue, where the pain was exactly coming from, the attending physician would admit the patient to the hospital and order X-rays of the upper gastrointestinal series, the only diagnostic tool available radiologically, to be done the following morning. This does not happen in modern-day medicine where everything will be done on outpatient basis. So the following morning, after overnight fasting, the patient would be sent to the radiology department, where the patient would undergo X-rays of the upper gastrointestinal series. A series of X rays would be taken as suggested by the name, starting from the esophagus, stomach, duodenum, and upper portion of small intestine after drinking a large cup of a liquid contrast material. If you take X-rays without contrast material, you cannot see anything.

This procedure is what I call "torture" not only to the radiologist who performs the procedure but also to the patient who has to go through the procedure. For both the patient and the radiologist, the room that the procedure is being done has to be called "torture chamber." They will all agree with me 100 percent. First, let's talk about the radiologist. Because he has to wear a gown which contains thick layers of lead, covering almost his entire body from neck to ankle, to protect himself from X-ray exposure. It is his lucky day if he picks up the responsible lesion in several trials, but if he does not, the torture for both patient and the doctor will last a lot longer. As a result, many of my radiologist colleagues suffer from low back problem, some of whom ended up having a back surgery and ultimately being forced to have an early and unplanned retirement. And second, let's talk about the patient. First thing in the next morning, the patient will be sent to the torture chamber, where he will be confined until the procedure is complete and the radiologist says the patient can be released. At the beginning of the procedure, the patient has to swallow a thick white mucuslike liquid as many times as the "torturer" tells him to do. There is no mercy from this torturer who continues to make the poor patient swallow this distasteful white liquid until he gets a satisfactory result.

Now with the result of the upper gastrointestinal series, it is the attending physician's destiny or decision to treat the patient with something. But with what? The best weapon among medical treatment has to be diet—the porridge made out of rice. Actually, it should have no salt, absolutely no salt, and should not be spicy at all. It should have no taste at all. As far as I can remember, the one and only medication that was available to the doctor at that era was the menthol-smelling thick white liquid called Amphojel, which is basically the same as Maalox or Mylanta, also known as antacid. The nurse comes in and gives one teaspoonful of this white stuff three or four times a day. This was how we treated a patient who was suspected to have peptic ulcer disease.

In modern-day medicine, everything will be done on outpatient basis. The moment a patient complains of epigastric or upper abdominal pain, depending on the urgency, either the patient will be sent to the emergency room for an emergency upper gastrointestinal endoscopy or be scheduled to have elective upper gastrointestinal endoscopy. The moment the gastroenterologist looks inside our stomach, he makes the diagnosis right away and comes up with a specific treatment plan, whether surgical or medical. If we decide to treat the patient medically, i.e., with medication, we have so many extremely efficient medications available to us in modern medicine. Pepcid is one of those, which is the focus of our discussion at the end of this chapter.

Now let us talk a bit about diabetes.

About the same time, forty or so years ago, it was not that difficult to make a diagnosis of diabetes compared to peptic ulcer disease. But the problem was the treatment of diabetes, which was more difficult than peptic ulcer disease. If you see a patient complaining of fatigue and sudden weight loss or gain associated with three big Ps which are the typical clinical features of diabetes—polyuria which means urinating a lot and more frequently, polydipsia which means drinking water a lot, and polyphagia which means eating a lot—you can make the diagnosis easily even before you do blood and urine tests, which will confirm the diagnosis afterward. Then the headache starts. It is big headache of the doctors. Because there are not many medicines to treat, only a few but very expensive.

Last and the third, let's talk about the speed. We have no reason to eat fast. But if you look around, you will find many people who eat fast, sometimes too fast. If you look at animals, most of them or maybe all of them eat fast until they reach a point where they do not need to eat anymore. It might be a good subject to have a research done why all the animals eat fast. Furthermore, it would be more interesting if someone does a research on human nature regarding the difference between someone who eats fast and someone who eats slow. We humans, unlike animals, have no reason to eat fast. We control our own speed. And yet among people, we can divide two groups of people—people who eat fast and people who eat slowly.

This is my question: "Why do some of us eat so fast even though there is absolutely no reason to do that?" Why? Why? Sometimes, a person like me who eats extremely slow eats real fast when and if I have a reason to eat fast. But majority of the time, if there is no reason to hurry, I eat extremely slow, sometimes super slow.

We can see there are two groups of people—who eat fast and who eat slow, when we eat hard candies and ice cubes. One group of people exhibits that the moment they drop a hard candy into their mouth, they break up the candy right away into million pieces with loud noise and swallow it down. It takes only a few seconds for the candy to disappear from their mouth. The same thing happens with ice cube. Why do they have to break up an ice cube into million pieces? It takes only a few seconds also to disappear. And the second group, the people who eat a candy slow and may take forever to finish one "stupid" candy. It stays in the mouth and melts away microscopically, one molecule of the candy at a time. The same thing happens with ice cube also. The ice cube stays in these people's mouths forever, one water molecule at a time until it melts down. And finally it disappears.

Ask yourself where do you belong. I hope all of you say you belong to the second group. Why? Because I am concerned about your precious stomach. Why? Then which stomach will last longer and healthier between the two, fast eater or slow eater? This is one of the big reasons why I'm writing this book to help you recognize the truth.

Definitely, the second group's stomach will last longer and healthier for sure. If you are a fast eater and agree with me, it is never too late to change for you and your stomach. Please change and join the second group. That's where we should all belong to live long and healthy.

So far, I have listed the three main culprits that can impact our stomach negatively. I would like to add a few more, something that we are all aware of, and then move on to the conclusion of this chapter.

Unfortunately, there is something called "stress" that can hurt our stomach. We are living under a lot of stress, probably under an enormous amount of stress. We are facing a tremendously harsh competition than the previous generations—nationally, internationally, socially, personally, and at home. Stress is everywhere. We cannot hide from it. We cannot avoid it. I do not have to explain it in detail because we are all under so much stress. And always, my stress, my headache, is much bigger than yours.

Unfortunately, there is also something called "cigarettes" that can give significant damage to our stomach. Among us, we have friends who smoke and cannot quit. It is one on my list of "the world's seven wonders." Among us, there are many who do not want to live long and healthy, and furthermore, there are many who want to cut short our precious life. I'm wondering why. Why can't some of us quit smoking? Why?

Unfortunately, there is also something called "alcohol" that can hurt our stomach. Among us, we have friends who drink excessively and are unable to control the impulse. This is also one on my list of the world's seven wonders. I'm wondering why. Why can't some of us quit alcohol? Why?

If we summarize all these together, we will come to realize that we—specifically our stomachs—are under attack by the enemies of the stomach, which are salty, spicy, and garlic-rich food; large meal; fast-eating habit; stress; cigarettes; and alcohol. In addition to these, we have one more important one that is waiting for us. It is probably the worst news of all—aging. Degenerative changes will make every single thing listed above worse, much worse.

These are the reasons why we have to take Pepcid, the guardian of humanity. No, it is the guardian of our stomach. Take one before you go to bed. Take one aspirin in the morning, just before or after breakfast or with a cup of milk if you are in a hurry. Take one Pepcid or acid controller before you go to bed please.

Enjoy your food as much as you can and to the limit but protect your stomach, the most abused organ in our body, at all costs, actually almost as little as no cost by taking one acid controller, i.e., Pepcid, before you go to bed from Costco if you consider the enormous benefit you get by taking one pill.

Before moving to the next chapter, I'd like to mention a little about the human history and recent occurrence of the fight or struggle against peptic ulcer disease caused by the acid that is produced by our own stomach. If you put your own or someone else's stomach fluid onto your skin, you will receive at least a second-degree burn, the same burn caused by the sun. You can easily imagine how strong the acidity our own stomach is producing inside our body, which is assaulting our stomach day in and day out, even while we are sleeping.

When I was graduating from medical school almost half of a century ago, the only medicine available was something called Amphojel. I have no idea how the doctors treated or managed peptic ulcer disease before my generation. Maybe with milk?

Apparently, we humans have been suffering from peptic ulcer disease ever since we were created by God thousands, thousands, and thousands of years ago. But the one and only medicine available to us to fight against the powerful stomach acid was Amphojel.

Now I'm introducing brief summaries of three groups of anti-ulcer medications that are available to us. First is antacid, such as Amphojel, Mylanta, Maalox, Rolaids, etc. Second is histamine H_2 receptor antagonists, such as Tagamet (cimetidine), Zantac (ranitidine), Pepcid (famotidine), and Axid (nizatidine). Third is proton-pump inhibitor, such as Prilosec (omeprazole), Nexium (esomeprazole), Protonix (pantoprazole), and Dexilant (dexlansoprazole).

The criteria that I choose in the selection of strong defense against peptic ulcer disease is the same as when I choose the best exercise for our health. First of all, it has to be effective. Second, the cost has to be reasonable. Third, it has to be readily available. It has to be easy to obtain. Due to the first criteria, the first group was eliminated without hesitation. Due to the second and third criteria, the third group was eliminated. So I choose one of the second group, which is an acid controller, also known as Pepcid, specifically from Costco.

Now let's talk about a recent occurrence with Zantac. We all know that when a medicine is developed and marked by a company, after ten years, any company is legally allowed to make the same medicine. But it is illegal to use the same name, which becomes generic. In the case of Zantac, "acid reducer" is the generic version, which is produced by Costco.

In September of this year 2019, the United States Food and Drug Administration (FDA) announced that some of the generic Zantacs were found to "contain a nitrosamine impurity called nitrosodimethylamine (NDMA) at low level. NDMA is classified as a probable human carcinogen (a substance that could cause cancer) based on results from laboratory tests. NDMA is a known environmental contaminant and found in water, and foods, dairy products, and vegetable." And the FDA already took action and removed those generic Zantacs from the market and announced that the generic Zantacs do not contain NDMA, including acid reducer, on which Costco took action already to remove from over the counter entirely. "FDA is not calling for individual to stop taking ranitidine at this time; however, patients taking prescription ranitidine who wish to discontinue use should talk to their health care professional about other treatment. People taking OTC ranitidine could consider using other OTC medicine approved for their condition."

This is exactly what I did to myself and my patients. I gave the choice to change to other equally effective, readily available, and reasonably cheap one, which is Pepcid, also known as acid controller in Costco.

CHAPTER 8

Black Madonna

There are numerous artistic expressions depicting Maria, the mother of Jesus. Typically, the most famous one is the *Pietà* created by Michelangelo in St. Peter's Basilica of the Vatican City. Among those arts, some are expressed in color black. This Black Madonna has an interesting reason why it is black.

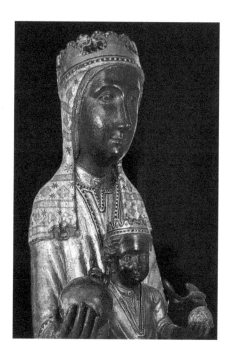

From the biggest city of Spain, present and past, Barcelona, about an hour drive, we can visit the tall and dangerous-looking rocky mountain range called Montserrat. Usually, when you go to Spain in a group, the tour company would schedule to visit this famous tourist attraction, Montserrat rocky mountain range, on Sunday morning. And after lunch, you would then go to the Gaudí House-Museum in Barcelona in the afternoon. So in order to digest this busy Sunday morning, you have to move fast.

To be able to attend the Sunday mass at ten o'clock in the morning and listen to and enjoy the world-famous boys' choir after the mass, you have to leave the hotel at eight o'clock in the morning. By the time you arrive at the church—I do not remember the exact time—it is already jam-packed inside. The big church has no empty seats but standing room only, and only just for a few. After the choir, you have to go and stand in a long line to meet this famous Black Madonna on the top of the church in a small chapel.

There is a good reason why so many people want to meet this lady with the boy Jesus. Probably, this is the main reason why so many people come to this place to meet the lady. In the early days of Christianity after the death of Jesus, St. Mark came to Spain to spread the good news. When he finished his mission and retuned to Jerusalem, he gave this Black Madonna to the people of Spain. But no one knew who was the sculptor. It is carved on a wood, with the mother sitting on the chair and the Son is standing in front of her and giving blessings to the people. With the passing of time, the color turned from a wooden color to black. No one painted it with black. The color changed by itself with time. Her right hand is holding a tennis ball-sized globe, and her left hand is empty. But this empty left hand is the one that gives us the miracles that we are praying, holding this famous hand. When we hold this empty left hand and pray, the miracle will come to us, whatever it may be.

But this statue mysteriously disappeared, and people forgot about the existence of St. Mark's gift of God's love. After hundreds of years passed, it reappeared the same way it disappeared. When a young shepherd was sleeping with his herds on the mountain, he noticed that a bright light was shining out from a small cave. He found the long-lost wooden statue of the Black Madonna in the cave and brought it to the village.

It was kept at the church of the village, but the people of the village started noticing the miracle that the statue showed. In medieval period, when people pray in front of the statue for the safe return of young sons or husbands from a war abroad or overseas expeditions and for the speedy recovery of sick members of families, numerous miracles happened. More people came not only from nearby villages but also as far from other neighboring European countries.

When Napoleon was in power, he decided to liberate and/or occupy and conquer Egypt from Turkish occupation. On the way to Egypt, he was going to stop by this village. The news that Napoleon was going to march past the village spread out to the people of the village, especially among the leaders, whose headaches got bigger and bigger and also heavier and heavier because what if Napoleon wanted to see it or Napoleon wanted to borrow it, saying he wanted to show the Black Madonna to his people back in Paris or all over the France and never returned it, then who would go and tell him to give it back without risking their life? But if they refused to give him, he would come and take it away by force anyway. So they came up with a brilliant idea. They decided to hide the statue somewhere no one knew and then told everybody that somebody, like a thief, stole it away.

Indeed, Napoleon came and sent his men to see if he could see the statue himself. They returned to Napoleon empty-handed and reported that it was stolen and missing.

Again, after a while, time had come for the statue to return to where it used to be. But there was one concern among the elderly, the leaders of the village. What if Napoleon came on the way back after hearing that the wooden statue came back to her place? Or what if another conqueror or strong figure came to the village, demanding to "borrow" it for his own satisfaction or for his own people's satisfaction? So they decided to make another statue, which is almost identical that no one could tell the difference. Of course, the real one was hiding somewhere deep in the mountain in a cave, where no one could see it anymore. So no one knows where the real one is.

In the beginning, as with the real one, the color was a wooden one, then gradually turned to black, like the real one as years passed by. Yes, since then, the one people, including myself, are praying in front of is not real. It is the fake one. But the very strange thing is that, as people continued to pray to the fake one, miracles continued to occur.

For several hundred years since then, how many people came to this wooden fake statue and pray? Astronomical? Yes, I'm sure it is more than the number of the stars in the sky. So many people came and went. Every one of them wanted to hold her left hand and pray. That's exactly what I did too.

Again, she is protected by a bulletproof plastic panel, like the *Pietà*, except her left hand so that people can hold her hand while praying.

Before moving on to the next chapter, there is one thing I have to make clear. It is an absolutely incorrect statement when people say many times that Catholics pray to the holy mother of Jesus. We Catholics never pray to her for miracle. We only pray to God for miracle, only God, no one else. Furthermore, we never pray to the saints, such as St. Peter or St. Paul, but only to ask for their help to move God to our direction. The only one we pray to for miracle is God the Almighty. By the way, the holy mother is one of the saints. Precisely speaking, we are praying to God the Almighty, no one else. And we are asking her to tell him what we need or what we want. Because she is the best lobbyist to move God toward us.

I remember so well that when I was little, if I wanted to have the same toy that my best friend had, instead of asking directly to my dad, I would convince my mom first. Then my mom would tell my dad what I wanted. Then my dad would never refuse or decline. My dad always listened to my mom. This is one of many mysteries of mine that I do not understand. I learned that trick when I was very little. That's exactly what I'm doing and all the Catholics are doing. Tell her first, and then she tells him what exactly I need. Then most of the time, he does not refuse, probably and hopefully all the time.

It sounds like we are praying to her, but the truth is we are praying to God, hoping he listens to this amazing lady and gives us what we want or what we need. Because we know so well that the one who allows the miracle to us is him, not her.

Even though I learned that trick when I was very little, I still do not know or understand the reason why it works so well. I still do not understand the mechanism how. To the best of my knowledge, I can think of two reasons.

First, God must be too busy to listen to my problem. God must be very busy taking care of other people whose pains are much bigger and worse than mine. There must be more desperate people in this world than I am. He is so busy and tied up with those people that he does not have enough time to listen to my problem. Second, God gave us free will as well as consequences. Yes, he is watching us. But he is waiting until the time comes. He is not even twitching or blinking when we are in trouble, asking for help. That is the contract we were given. He signed the contract with us and does not want to break the contract each time we ask. At this crucial moment, we bring the best lobbyist we ever have, who is the mother of his Son. I'm sure he will twitch his facial muscle. He is so fair. If I choose to do something good, something good will happen to me. If I choose to do something bad intentionally or unintentionally, something bad will happen to me. After I did something bad and yet I want something good to happen to me, will he listen? What if you are in his shoes, are you going to listen and act? But it is still a mystery to me.

Of course, we Catholics, like anyone else, pray to God directly, one on one, pleading, asking, demanding, sometimes even threatening, and so on. That's what I do many times. I go directly to him, who has the ability and the power to give the miracle I need. Why do I have to go through someone else? Why bother? It's wasting my time and energy. So I go directly to him. But nothing happens. Then I pray to Jesus, his Son. Same thing! No response. Nothing happens. He must be busy like his dad. And finally, I ask her to tell my problem, my difficulty, to him or his Son. How come he or his Son listens to her? I learned this trick long after I became a Catholic. It took a long time to learn this trick. First of all, I myself want to take care of my problem. If I can take care of my problem, why do I need help from others, including God? I do my best to solve my problem.

Third, if and when I have a problem that I cannot handle, I choose to talk to God the Almighty and the one and only directly, one on one, from man to God. If he does not respond, then I talk to his Son. His Son does not respond either. Both of them must be very busy. Then who else? I talk to her. And I receive the answer.

So I have a big suggestion to everyone. It does not matter what religion you have. When you have a problem and need to talk to God, talk to him first, then his Son. If there is no answer, go and talk to her and ask her to tell either one of them and then wait and see what happens.

Here, this is the second half of the Hail Mary, my favorite. To me, the first half is not as important as the second half, although the entire Hail Mary is important. The second half is as follows: "Holy Mary, mother of God, pray for us, sinners, now and at the hour of our death. Amen."

She is the one who prays to God for us to go to the better place and buries us in her heart. We do not ask her to make a miracle for us, but we ask her to give us a small favor to relay our trouble, our problem, to him. How can he send our souls to a place where we do not want to go, a place that is worse than heaven, the so-called hell, when she buries our soul in her heart?

CHAPTER 9

Aspirin

After I finished my residency training, I joined a group practice. One morning, there was an old woman who was admitted through the emergency room because of a massive stroke, with paralysis on one side. I forgot which side was affected. She had been seen by an emergency room physician, and the diagnosis was well established by the clinical finding as well as CAT scan and lab results.

According to my judgment, her prognosis was so bad that I planned to discharge her within a few days and called her daughter and set up an appointment to discuss the long-term plan. But about three days later, the patient showed a definite sign of improvement. To me, I felt like I was witnessing some kind of a miracle. But miracle did happen right in front of my eyes, which made me a true believer of a miracle of some kind. Five or six days later, she was able to move her affected side with the help of physical therapy and began to speak. After ten days, by the time she was discharged, she was able to stand up and walk. Even though she was able to walk, she was discharged on a wheelchair due to hospital policy.

Before I discharged her, I had a lengthy talk to see if I can come up with a something that might be responsible for her alleged miracle of sort. Apparently, she had serious multiple medical problems, for which she was prescribed more than the usual medications. Among those was one particular medicine that got my attention. It came out as one of the over-the-counter medicines. It was aspirin.

Because she was suffering from a severe case of degenerative osteoarthritis, she was given and tried all kinds of NSAIDS (nonsteroidal antiinflammatory drugs). But nothing worked, and none of them was effective, except aspirin. Actually, aspirin is at the bottom of the totem pole among the family of NSAIDS in terms of effectiveness, especially for pain control. Aspirin would be at the bottom of all medicines for pain control. But whether you believe it or not, aspirin was the only medicine that works for her arthritic pain. And she was taking a rather unusual number of aspirin pills a day. I do not remember the exact number she was taking. So in my opinion, aspirin is the one. Aspirin is the main reason she recovered from her massive stroke.

We, including myself, who have no reason to take aspirin should take aspirin also. Even a healthy person who does not have any medical indication whatsoever should take aspirin like this old lady, but not as much as or as often as she was taking. The reason is when we get older, our blood tends to become thicker than normal for various reasons. Thus, we have to thin the blood to some extent to prevent thrombus formation inside the blood vessels, particularly in the arterial side, and prevent the thrombus to become a blockage locally or become emboli to move from the original site to any of the distant part of our body—such as lung, brain, or heart—and become the cause of pulmonary embolism, stroke, or heart attack, which are often fatal or can cripple our range of activity and thus diminish our quality of life.

We can just take one baby aspirin only a day. One baby aspirin (81 milligrams) is one-fourth amount of an adult aspirin (325 milligrams). I recommend all of us to take one baby aspirin in the morning just before or after our breakfast. If you are too busy to have your breakfast, then drink a cup of milk. The side effect is little to minimal because you are taking such a low dose. And think about the benefit.

But there is a group of people who should not take any aspirin. For example, someone who is already taking one of the NSAIDS, especially one who suffered from upper gastrointestinal bleeding after taking any of the NSAIDS; someone who have blood dyscrasia, such as leukemia or pernicious anemia or thrombocytopenia, which means low platelet in the blood; and someone who is going to have a dental procedure, such as tooth extraction, or invasive procedure, such as upper or lower gastrointestinal endoscopy with potential biopsies of polyps or suspicious lesion anywhere in the gastrointestinal tract, etc.

Oftentimes, many of my cardiologist colleagues tell me that they advise their patients with heart problems to take a handful of aspirin immediately, if and when they develop chest pains and/or shortness of breath before they call for an ambulance. You are not going to see this kind of advice or recommendation in any textbooks or journals.

So when I wake up in the morning, before I start my day, I take one baby aspirin and go out.

Among those who take aspirin already for one reason or another, these are the benefits of taking a baby aspirin a day.

After a massive heart attack, the person survives. That is because the person was taking aspirin. If a person had a mild heart attack who should have been a victim of a massive heart attack, that is because again the person was taking aspirin. Also, after a massive stroke, the person survives. That's because the person was taking aspirin. If a person had a mild stroke who should have been a victim a massive stroke, that's because again the person was taking aspirin. So many people take aspirin and don't know what aspirin does to them. Thus, they do not appreciate what aspirin does to their body.

And these are other examples of why aspirin is being underappreciated most of the time or at all. There are many people, like the following examples, among the stroke victims. It is literally impossible to collect the data, as no one can give you numbers. But this is true.

But there were many researches done in long-term, double-blind studies by national level in European countries and America or by an organization like the World Health Organization which showed statistically significant differences between those group who took aspirin and placebo. Thus, it has been a long time ago since the FDA approved to use aspirin for the prevention of both stroke and heart attack. We all know that we can buy baby aspirin over the counter without a doctor's prescription in drugstores. Many of you have made the decision to take this amazing miracle pill already.

So practically, it is an ongoing fact that there are many people currently taking one baby aspirin a day who are living healthy without being struck by a stroke or heart attack at this hour and who are direct beneficiaries of the aspirin effect.

Oftentimes, you might have heard about this kind of people among your relatives or close friends, a victim of stroke but never recognized by the patient themselves, families, or even caretakers. It is so mild that it comes and goes, being never recognized. Sometimes, the tongue feels numb. Then the feeling comes back. And back and forth. Sometimes, part of the visual field goes dark and then comes back. And back and forth. Sometimes, the tip of the fingers or the toes goes numb. Then the feeling comes back. And back and forth. Sometimes, a person slips or drops their spoon or chopsticks for no reason. And back and forth. Oftentimes, this is an early warning signal of an upcoming massive stroke. So many of the massive stroke victims remember such episodes after or if they survive. We call this transient ischemic attack, also known as ministroke. But I'd like to call this microstroke. Calling it "mini" seems very unscientific to me. It is something we are unable to see with the naked eye and only able to see under the microscope. To me, "micro" sounds more scientific than "mini."

In such a condition of imminent danger of a massive magnitude, it is aspirin that will protect us by minimizing the outcome of strokes from massive to moderate, from moderate to mild, from mild to micro, and from micro to nothing happened. How wonderful what aspirin does to our body! What a silent hero! Aspirin prevents stroke from happening in advance.

There are many people, like the following examples, among heart attack victims. But it is literally impossible to collect the data. I cannot give you exactly how many. Simply, there are many, but we cannot put it into numbers how many of us are the beneficiaries of this wonderful medicine. Oftentimes, you might have heard about this kind of people among your relatives or close friends, victim of a heart attack but never recognized by the patient themselves, families, or even caretakers. It is so mild that it comes and goes, being never recognized. Sometimes, it feels like a real chest pain of heart, but sometimes not. Sometimes it is so mild that you ignore it. Sometimes, it does not feel like a chest pain of heart attack that you mix it up with indigestion, gastritis, esophagitis, bronchitis, etc.

So up until not too long ago, people thought and called it acute indigestion syndrome if someone dies suddenly with a massive heart attack at a dinner table. Many times, this is a kind of early warning sign of upcoming massive heart attack. Many of the victims of massive heart attack remember such episodes after or if they survive. We call this kind of heart attack silent myocardial infarction or silent heart attack. We may call this "silent," but it will never be silent at all soon after or eventually.

This is what aspirin is doing to our body, minimizing the result of heart attack from massive to mild, from mild to silent, and from silent to nothing happened. How wonderful what aspirin does to our body! What a silent hero!

Initially, aspirin was born to this world as one of the antipyretic and analgesic agents. Mostly as an antipyretic, we desperately needed a good medicine for fever, not only for the babies but also for the grown-ups. But currently, the FDA approved it for more than a few more indications other than its initial purpose.

There are many medicines that became more famous because of their "side effect" than the initial and original purpose of the medication itself. Two best examples are Viagra and Rogaine. Both of them are developed initially for the treatment of hypertension. Somehow, they turned out to have remarkable effectiveness for other conditions. Both of them made a fortune to their company and stockholders.

Anyway, for the younger generations, they do not need to take aspirin. But the older generations who start to exhibit the signs of degenerative changes externally should take one baby aspirin a day, along with Pepcid.

After all these explanations and evidences of why we should take aspirin, if there are certain people who think that they don't have to take aspirin, how do we describe these people's mind and behavior? Self-destructive or suicidal? But I do not mind whatever the reason behind it.

Once again, I strongly recommend aspirin to everybody, except to those who should not take it. No matter how healthy a person is, if you are over sixty years old, you should take aspirin. A dose of 81 milligrams of baby aspirin, which is one-fourth of an adult dose, is very tiny so that it is very easy to swallow.

Simply because I strongly recommended aspirin, I have not received anything—cash or any favor—from the aspirin company. Not even a single penny. None of my families works for the aspirin company. It's the same with Pepcid, i.e., acid controller.

CHAPTER 10

Hepburn

We have a very fond memory of two Hepburns who are not with us anymore. We, i.e., the old generation, remember well Audrey (1929–1993) and Katharine (1907–2003). We can see both of them at TCM (Turner Classic Movies) channel if we are lucky.

In this chapter, I'm going to talk about Katharine. I do not need to explain how good or excellent she was as an actress because I'm not in that business. But just the fact that, in the history of the Academy Awards, she was nominated twelve times and received the Best Actress Award four times tells us how good she was. Although in the twenty-first century, a person whose name is Meryl Streep broke the world record of Academy Awards nominations with thirteen times, the winning record of four is still unbroken and intact.

Every year by the end of February, there is an Academy Awards ceremony. In early January, the Academy announces the nominees. Then the entertainment world becomes noisy and even the loudest on the night of the ceremony when the winners are announced. This year, Leonardo DiCaprio is one of the nominees for the Best Actor Award. He was nominated several times before but never won. Always, there was a dark horse, who was not so good-looking but with brilliant acting skills, who took away the award from DiCaprio. There are more than several of these so-called handsome and commercially very successful actors that never won the Oscars' leading actor at this time. You know who they are. We have known Leonardo since he was little from TV, but ever since he became famous in the movie *Titanic*, I saw every movie he starred. But I was a bit concerned if he might be one of the many superstars who finish their career without winning the biggest award in their field. Like in sports, such as football, baseball, basketball, ice hockey, etc., especially golf. There are many excellent professional golfers who made tons of money by winning many tournaments other than majors but ended their career without winning majors. Once there was a famous golfer, whose other name was the best professional golfer, who never won a major. You know who I'm talking about. But I do not hear those negative comments anymore. I think many people in the media realized that it is always better being positive. In the public domain, positive always wins; by the same token, negative always loses.

Anyway, unlike other actors or actresses in those years, many became movie stars by accident. But it was Katharine's childhood dream to pursue an acting career. And she majored in acting in college, then went to Hollywood to be a star. Rarely do we see some people who not only are very successful in their field but also, at the same time, help and make others successful. She was one of them.

She helped John Wayne, who never won an Academy, to win an Academy just before he died. I like John Wayne. Not only he used to be my childhood hero because I grew up watching his Western movies back in Korea but also he invested all his hard-earned money into the movie industry. He had little money left when he died.

And she helped Henry Fonda, who also never won an Academy, to win an Academy. He watched from a hospital bed his daughter accepting the award on his behalf. In the movie *On Golden Pond*, not only did she help him win an Oscars but she also took one for herself.

But she had one big childhood psychological trauma. She was the one who found her younger brother dead, who hanged himself by mistake while practicing alone in a room a magic trick he learned from their father. The trauma must have been deep.

All through her life, she never put on any makeup, except only when she was in front of a camera while making movies. She never wore expensive clothes when she was not making movies so that not many people recognized her if she was in the crowd. She never gave any interviews with a reporter or talk show host, with only one exception.

After she got married in 1928 and then divorced in 1941, she never married again. And yet we all remember her famous relationship with Humphrey Bogart and that they loved each other but never got married. The two became lifelong friends while making the movie *Woman of the Year*. They remained friends until he died of lung cancer. She took care of him until the moment he died.

More than a few times before, I visited Boston to attend a continuing medical education course or other occasions. But few years ago, when I was making a schedule to go to Boston again, I added three more days to the schedule to visit the state of Maine, up to the northernmost part of America on that side next to Canada.

As soon as I arrived at the Logan Airport, I rented a car. First, I stopped by Cape Cod and visited Martha's Vineyard, where John F. Kennedy used to spend his summer vacation with his family. Then I drove north along the Atlantic coastline until I reached the state of Maine, specifically the Acadia National Park, which was my destination. Then I turned around to south, but not the same route. Instead of going down the Atlantic coast, I changed the direction a bit inland to the direction of the state of New Hampshire. I visited the Blue Mountain and the White Mountain.

Again, I realize that I'm not a literary major. I'm a scientist, a doctor. I cannot describe how beautiful and magnificent Acadia National Park was. The Blue Mountain and the White Mountain as well. For example, when I went to the Grand Canyon, in front of the grandness of God's magnificent creation, I felt the greatness at the bottom of my heart, not from my brain. How can I describe it with my tiny and limited brain? It is impossible. Simply, it's better to be honest and give up. You have to see it to believe it. When you are under a deep anesthesia by nature, time flies. Suddenly, you find yourself in the dark. Where did the sun disappear? You have to find a place to spend the night and calm down your mumbling stomach. I found a small town in the middle of nowhere with the help of GPS. I rushed to the town, hoping that there was a decent restaurant.

Katharine Hepburn had a secretary, also known as an assistant, who was almost like her own sister in almost their lifetime together. She went everywhere her boss went. They traveled together if the boss had to go out of town or out of the country for filming. The secretary was given two weeks of summer vacation. That was when she went back home and spent the time with her parents and sisters and brothers together because she traveled many of the places in and out of the country already with her boss. So when her secretary went home for two weeks every summer, her boss also went to the same town, but they're not together. She rented a suite at the local hotel a little bit away from the town and spent two weeks alone. Then she went back to New York and continued her work as usual. She spent most of her time reading books in her suite or walking on a trail. Occasionally, she appeared in a local restaurant and disappeared quietly.

When I checked into the hotel, suddenly, the lady at the front desk asked me a question. Actually, it was an offer that I could not decline. How could I? She said, "Do you want to have the suite where Katharine Hepburn used to stay? There is no extra charge." How could I refuse? How could anyone refuse? I was going to sleep in the same room where she, the one I admire the most, used to sleep in the past. I was going to read a book in the room as she did a long time ago, was I?

Katharine Hepburn never gave any interview with a reporter or any talk show host in her whole career, except on one occasion only. That was with Barbara Walters of ABC News. At the end of her interview, Barbara Walters asked her one important question: "Do you have Parkinson's?"

We do not know how long, but she seemed to have been shaking or nodding her head continuously for more than several years. Because I do not or cannot see her hands shaking, it is difficult to make the diagnosis 100 percent. At that crucial moment, I was anticipating that she was going to say either yes or an "I don't know" kind of response. But to my surprise, she did not disappoint anyone, including myself. Her answer was very simple; it was just one word—no. While she was looking at the interviewer eye to eye, she did not give any explanation whatsoever. That is the reason why I continue to *respect* her even now and more than ever.

CHAPTER 11

Sleep

I do not need to explain too much about sleep. Because we are all experts about sleep itself one way or another, whether we are a good sleeper or a bad sleeper. And there is nothing much to add to what we know already. We are experts about sleep because we sleep every night. We spend many hours of sleep every day without missing this valuable part of our life every single day, specifically every single night.

First of all, those people who do not have any problem, none whatsoever, with sleeping at night do not have to read this chapter. Why waste time? Just continue to do what you are doing and move on. Worry about this issue when you lose this blessing.

Like anyone else, I myself did not have this problem until not too long ago. Why bother? Sleep issue never bothered me until not too long ago. Now I have a serious problem with insomnia. Since I know what is the cause of my insomnia and, more importantly, I know how to take care of my insomnia, I'm going to share how to solve your insomnia.

This chapter is written for those who have a serious problem with falling asleep, the so-called insomnia. Like any other health issues, I'm going to mention how to solve the problem and give you the answer at the end of this chapter if you have a problem with sleeping. I understand and admit also that so many people are suffering from this issue and seeking the bad and wrong solutions of their own. I sincerely hope that more than many people find the solution that I offer in this chapter.

Anyway, whether you have a problem with sleeping or not, we have to sleep for almost one-fourth to one-third of our daily life, which means we spend one-fourth or one-third of our entire life with our eyes closed. Most recent study show that seven hours of sleep would be the most ideal. But in my opinion, although I'm not an expert in the area of sleep, six hours of sound sleeping should be more than enough. Anyway, it is hard to say one way or another because everyone has a different pattern of sleeping. I'll do my best to describe insomnia and, one thing for sure, to tell at the end of this chapter the solution for insomnia. I hope you agree and choose to follow my advice.

In terms of pattern of sleep, there are two extremes, and everybody falls somewhere in between.

One extreme is those people who go to bed and fall asleep immediately, and then until they wake up in the morning, they do not remember anything. The only thing they remember is the fact that they went to bed the night before. They do not remember anything, even though thieves broke into and cleaned up the entire house. I know several friends, couples, who go to bed as soon as they finish dinner at home. The only few exceptions for them to go to bed late would be when they have to attend a wedding reception, some kind of dinner party, etc. Yes, they are born to sleep. They are very happy, and they never regret the fact that they are in sleep more than one-third or a bit less than half of their lives doing nothing but sleeping. What a waste, but these are a bunch of people who are very happy, even though they do nothing but sleep for almost ten hours a day.

And now let's talk about the other extreme. I know only a few of this kind of people compared to the first group. I'm very happy that I know only a few of these people, not many. I'm introducing a small group of people who are on the other extreme. These people are the kind of people who do not sleep at night, not even during the day called "napping." I have seen a lot of patients suffering from insomnia. But this group of people are above and beyond the scope of insomnia. When they go to bed, their minds become clearer than before. Even though they close their eyes, their eyes are brighter than ever so that they have to open their eyes. Staying in bed for two or three hours without sleeping is becoming a so painful physical and psychological nightmare that falling asleep is ever more difficult. Then here comes the morning sun. At the age of sixty, this person does not remember that they had had any sleep any night or day all their life. This is a true story of one person's life, and I did not make up this story. And it is also true that there are hundreds, thousands, and millions of people in this world who are suffering from this so-called insomnia, not worse than the person described above but close to the person above.

I'm sure there will be a lot of people who are going tell themselves, "This is my story," or "I'm close to those people." So I'm going to talk about the cause and the seriousness of insomnia and, more importantly, the solution of insomnia at the conclusion of this chapter, as I always do and will be doing when dealing with health issues.

Before I go into the real pathological insomnia, let me briefly mention about "artificial" or "iatrogenic" or "man-made" insomnia. I myself used to be one of those who had to go through this kind of sleeping problem, i.e., sleep deprivation, when I was young. I'm assuming there are a lot of people who went through this "disease" and who are currently going through this problem. I recall all those sleep-deprived faces, including myself, who were preparing for the college entrance exam in Korea during the senior year of high school. Actually, the competition now must be much worse than when I was facing this challenge in the past. And more importantly, I always remember and respect those people who work at night. Especially those in the military who provide us, citizens of America, a good night sleep. Also those in the police department, in the correction department, in the fire department, in the hospital, in the auto company, and so on. They are the ones who do not have insomnia but have to stay awake to protect and to provide a better quality of life for the benefit of the rest of us. I myself used to belong to this group of people, so I understand what they are going through. We never forget those young ones who sacrifice their precious sleeps to provide the rest of us a good night sleep.

Now I'm going to go over those people who suffer from lack of sleep, i.e., insomnia, a pathological lack of sleep. These are the sleep-deprived people who are so desperate and willing to take even narcotics to solve their problem. It is relatively simple to explain the definition of insomnia. First, there are people who have difficulty in falling asleep and who have a hard time initiating sleep. Second, there are people who can fall asleep in the beginning but wake up in the middle of sleeping then have hard time going back to sleep.

There are many experts about insomnia who keep their mouth shut or mull when it comes to the solution to this illness. The reason might be that it is next to impossible to find the solution for insomnia. Then shall we go out and find the solution for insomnia together? If someone does have a better solution than what we are about to find out, let us know. Share your secret with us.

Not too long ago, in Seoul, South Korea, world-famous experts in insomnia gathered around and had a huge conference, i.e., symposium, about insomnia. And they went home empty-handed. Why? Even though I did not attend the meeting, I know they went home without any solution. If they found the solution, the entire world would be completely different by now. First and foremost, I would be a completely different person. I'm going to be happy and contented. I would be the most likeable human being in the entire universe. And if there will be thousands and thousands of people and millions and millions of people like me in this universe, how can there be any disputes among people, and how can there be wars among countries?

As a first step, why do we have difficulty in sleeping? What is the cause of insomnia? And furthermore, where did my insomnia come from? We have to reflect on ourselves first to find out what is the cause of your and my insomnia. But in general, let's find out what is the cause of insomnia. If we find the cause, then there is hope to find the solution for insomnia. At this point, someone can ask questions like these: "Why bother? Why do we waste our energy when we have the solution already? Don't you know we have something called sleeping pill? We can take one pill when we have a problem falling asleep. It's so simple!" Wow!

Actually, the truth is there is no medication specifically manufactured for the purpose of sleeping aid. Most of, if not all, the over-the-counter sleeping aids are antihistamines, which were manufactured for the treatment of allergies of our body, most commonly runny nose and itchy eyes. The major side effect of this group of medicine is drowsiness. There is no medicine specifically manufactured for the purpose of sleep per se. And the most commonly prescribed medicine for sleeping aid is benzodiazepines, which is an antianxiety agent and definitely not for sleeping. There are short-acting, intermediate-acting, and long-acting benzodiazepines. The most notoriously famous one, Valium, is a long-acting benzodiazepine. And the doctors are prescribing and choosing one of those short-acting benzos. To be honest with you, there is no sleeping pill per se. The sleeping pill prescribed and given by your doctor belongs to short-acting benzos, which are actually one of the short-acting antianxiety drugs. The so-called over-the-counter sleeping pills that you can buy without a doctor's prescription are antihistamines, which we take when we have allergies. If you read the side effects of these antihistamines, it says dizziness, drowsiness, etc. Kindly, it will say, "Do not drive cars or heavy machines after you take this medicine." Go Google.

Again, there is no such thing called sleeping pill, period! These antianxiety agents are excellent medicines for anxiety, but these have an addictive tendency if you like them. If you use these medicines long enough, your body will develop a resistance. Yes, if you like them, they will like you too. You cannot get away from them. They will not let you go anywhere. You have to stay with them, and they will stay with you. That's exactly what happened to Michael Jackson and Prince, with pain pills and sleeping pills. If you stay close to these medicines, they will stay close to you until you die. That's how much they love you. The "beauty," i.e., notoriety, of these medicines is once you are addicted to one of these, sooner or later, your body will develop a tolerance, i.e., resistance. Thus, your body demands more to achieve the same result, and so you need more and then even stronger ones. So the medicine demands to increase the amount, more and more and more. Eventually, you have to change the medicine to a stronger one. You have no choice. The medicine will choose the stronger one, not you. And the vicious cycle ensues and continues and never goes back and will only get worse. Initially, people start with the mildest benzo with the minimal amount. Then the amount goes up, followed by a change to a stronger one. Again, the amount goes up, then moves to a new and stronger one, and so on. Again, this is exactly what happened to Michael Jackson and Prince. You know the rest of the story and what happened to them.

When I go to Chicago, about thirty minutes before arrival, I pass the tip of Indiana, a city called Gary. That's the city where Michael Jackson was born. Whenever I pass Gary, Indiana, I think about him and pray for him real quick.

When I go to California, sometimes I visit a nice city called Hollywood. If I take a city tour in a minibus, it stops at many different places, and the tour guide, usually the driver, explains what the place is famous for. The bus stops in front of or at the back of houses where a famous movie star, singer, professional athlete, or comedian used to live or still is living. And the tour guide explains about the house and the entertainer. As one of the stops, the tour bus stops at a familiar house, and the tour guide asks, "Do any of you know whose house this is?" Then he explains, "This is Michael Jackson's house. He used to stay and live in this house when he comes to Hollywood. And when he died, he went to the emergency room in an ambulance through that gate."

I remember the gate, although I do not know whether it is the front or rear gate. I saw it so many times on TV, so many days and so many months and on and on and on. I remember the house and the gate. In my opinion, Michael Jackson is the best and the most talented entertainer of all time, the one and only. There was nobody like him before. There will be nobody like him in the future in the history of mankind. Sometimes, actually many times, I question God, the one and only, "If you gave Michael such a talent and such a voice that only you can give, why did you give him insomnia and pain? Why? What is your message? Among all the athletes, Michael Jordan would be always the same. There is no one like him before and after. He will not change. Why did you give Michael Jackson something that you did not give to the other MJ, Michael Jordan?"

Somehow, both of the two who I like so much have same first name. Both of them are known to us as MJ. Is it a coincidence or what?

Also, the doctors are prescribing antihistamine for sleep aid, but actually, you can buy it over the counter. But patients do not like antihistaminic sleep aid because antihistamines can give us drowsiness and dizziness after we take them. So people prefer benzos.

Again, sleeping pills are not the solution for insomnia. I do not know the mechanism of action of these medicines once they get into our system and how they work on our brain cells. You can check Google if you want to know. My main concern is whatever you take or whatever you do, as long as you achieve the goal which is to make you fall asleep, I have no problem. But my real concern is the addiction potential of these medicines. I do not want anyone to be a slave of anyone or anything. Like everyone else, I want to be free. I want to own myself. I do not want to be owned by something or someone other than me. Do you?

If you want to know about the addiction potential of benzos, just look at Michael Jackson. Once you become a slave of someone or something, you have to do whatever they tell you to do. There are many things like this which have an addiction potential, such as drugs, which we are discussing now. There are also alcohol, nicotine, gambling, food, etc. I do not want to be addicted to any of the above. I want to be free. I do not want to be controlled by somebody or something other than me.

From now on, I'm going to discuss about the cause and treatment of insomnia. This is not something that I created on my own. It is the same with other health issues, all the solutions of which are what I learned from the textbook, in the classroom, and from others.

In my opinion, which I hope you all agree, this is the best and one and only way to solve the problem of insomnia. If anyone has better idea, please share with me and us. This is the best and the most accurate explanation of the cause and treatment of insomnia, which is very simple—we have to be tired to have a good sleep, both physically and psychologically. Our body and our muscles have to be tired, and our brain has to be tired. To put it the other way, if we are not tired on both, there is no good sleep.

I gave you the answer first, and then here comes the cause. If we solve the problem of being tired or being not tired, then the problem of insomnia will not be with us any longer. To make a long story short, the cause of insomnia is being not tired, and the treatment of insomnia is getting tired physically and psychologically.

When I'm talking about being tired, there are two aspects—being tired physically and being tired psychologically. These two things have to happen at the same time—meaning, together. If only one of the above is tired and the other is not, then there will be no good sleep.

To give you the answer for being tired physically, there is one and only way to do it, which is exercise, which I explained in the chapter "Exercise, the Most Important of All." If I come up with a formula, it is as follows: good night sleep = physical fatigue + psychological fatigue. Does anyone have any better idea other than the above? Please share with me and us.

To explain about being tired psychologically, unfortunately, it is the psychiatrist's, psychologist's, minister's, priest's area, not mine. I mean they are better than I am.

When you are thinking about physical and psychological fatigue simultaneously, the good example of this phenomenon would be a young cadet in West Point or a young man or young girl in a basic training camp or people like us on a trip to Alaska or Europe.

And another talking point, insomnia is not a simple problem. It is much worse than the common cold or even high blood pressure or sugar problem. For those problems such as hypertension or diabetes, we have many ways to deal with them as listed before, either medicinal approach or nonmedicinal approach or both, with minimal side effects in terms of being addictive in nature. But as far as insomnia is concerned, in my opinion, we have no other choice but only the nonmedicinal approach.

Please do not try to solve insomnia with pills or medicines. There is no pill for insomnia. You already know what the nonmedicinal approach is, which is exercise. We cannot kill this monster with a sleeping pill. If you, whether you are a doctor or a patient, think you can solve this problem by just taking a pill or two, you are making a big mistake. You have a big problem. Especially if you are a physician and you think you can solve this issue of your patients with a medicine, think again. Did your professor teach you that you can kill this monster with a pill? If your professor did not teach you that way, then it is you who are raising this monster. Change your mind right now. It is never too late.

Yes, we can kill this monster with short-acting, intermediate-acting, long-acting benzos, and, furthermore, stronger ones that Michael Jackson took or was given with intramuscularly or intravenously. I am sure Michael Jackson started taking or was given pills by mouth, then was switched to intramuscular, and ultimately to intravenous. That's what he did. That's what his doctor did. He went to the emergency room by ambulance with an IV line on his arm. But look at the outcome. Once we kill this monster with pills, then we are next. We get killed by these medicines, these so-called sleep aids. Why do we go to the wrong road that's proven to be wrong?

In terms of medicinal approach, there is only one exception. It is melatonin. It is used only for the geriatric population. Young people do not need this medicine. The pituitary gland in our brain produces melatonin when the sun goes down. The darkness around us when the sun goes down stimulates the pituitary glands to produce the hormone called melatonin. That's why we feel sleepy with darkness because of this substance. So melatonin is needed only by those people who cannot produce enough to make them feel sleepy. I do not mind the elderly trying this medicine. If it helps, continue taking it. If not, quit taking it. This medicine, melatonin, does not have an addictive nature, which means it's safe to take and safe to discontinue.

It is not my area of expertise, but it is something we have to think about. I'm not a psychiatrist, but we need to think about insomnia as a psychological perspective. Many of the psychiatric illnesses do have insomnia as part of their symptoms and, at times, as one of the warning signs of their illness. Only as a tip of the iceberg will you suffer from insomnia. In other words, many of the psychiatric illnesses start with insomnia and continues as part of the illnesses.

For example, a twenty-year-old young man came to the emergency room, escorted by two police officers because he was threatening to kill his family, claiming that his family was poisoning his food. This was the first episode of his long history of schizophrenia, a paranoid type. But his acute episodes were always preceded by two or three nights in a row of not sleeping or being unable to sleep.

Also, a twenty-year-old young woman came to a psychiatrist's office, escorted by her parents because she locked herself in her room, not eating, drinking, and sleeping. Her parents said whenever she went into her episode of depression, she was not sleeping for two or three nights in a row. That's how they could tell their daughter was in an acute episode of her mental illness.

Not only with significant psychiatric illnesses, like the above examples, but also with a little bit of emotional disturbances, such as extreme anger or anxiety or a bit of stress at work or at home, do we not sleep. We suffer from insomnia.

So in order for us to take care of the problem, i.e., insomnia, it would be dead wrong if the doctor prescribes sleeping pills instead of searching for the root cause of insomnia psychologically and physically. For the physical aspect of insomnia, to find the solution, I gave you the answer already. For the psychological aspect of insomnia, to find the solution, you have to find the reason and then ultimately you have to find the solution, with the help of a psychologist or a psychiatrist if necessary. Always we have to think deep if we have a problem with sleeping to see whether this could be the tip of something serious down under or a warning signal. Sometimes, due to something called stress, we can have insomnia.

By now, you know very well how to handle your problem. Instead of looking for the "magic" pill, you have to look at yourself. In any case of the examples listed above, you have to sit down and spend some time to reflect on yourself. You have to question yourself, "What could be the reason for my insomnia?" If you think it requires to talk to someone or an expert, do not hesitate. You have to do it. But like anything else in life, you are the one who knows better than anyone else what your problem is. Usually, you are the one who can find the solution, the answer, or the key to your problem. Don't even think that a pill will make your insomnia go away. If you are looking for the answer somewhere else other than yourself, you are one of the millions who are looking for the answer at wrong places. So when you think that you have an ongoing difficulty in decent sleeping, you have to look at what is going on in your mind. At the same time, you have to look at the other side and ask yourself, "Am I working out enough?" If you have a problem with sleeping, look at these two areas. Please do not look at anywhere else. If you do, you know what will happen to you. This is not threatening from me. I have no reason to threaten you, my fellow human being. I'm telling you the truth.

A sleeping pill, also known as sleep aid, especially one of the benzos, is not something that helps us to sleep well. It acts like helping us initially and makes us feel so wonderful that we have found the solution for our problem. But sooner or later, it will become our worst nightmare and easily will destroy us. The sleep aid becomes our nightmare.

Yes, a narcotic painkiller will make sure to kill our pain and make sure we feel wonderful and pain free. But sooner or later, it will become our worst nightmare and easily will kill us. Like the name, a painkiller will kill our pain, but we are the next. It will kill us.

Sleeping pills and narcotics have strong addiction potentials. They help us solve our difficulty, acting as if they are a problem solver, like a superhero. But sooner or later, they become something bigger than us and something more important than we are within ourselves. What a tragedy! It is pills who decide our future, not us. What a tragedy! They make us lie to and cheat at our family and our friends. Ultimately, we cheat ourselves. They make us steal money and ultimately make us kill others for not a whole lot of money. But we are the ones who make the decision. We make the choice, no one else. When we were born, we were given free will from God the Almighty. So we are the ones that make all the choices and all the decisions. We are the ones that make the choices with our free will. We get the credit if the result is good. But if the result is bad, we blame God. We blame everything to God if we do not get what we want.

I have a small question to my fellow physicians. Why we are not telling the truth about benzos and narcotics to our beloved patients so that they make the right choices? All of us, both as physicians and patients, have to look deep inside ourselves whether we are making the right choices, not the wrong decisions.

Now let's turn to the general aspects of a good sleep. Most of us already know. We have to go to bed before midnight. The most ideal time to go to bed is between ten and eleven, never after twelve. Sleeping after midnight would not be a good one. Unless we have a good and legitimate reason to go to bed after midnight, we should always go to bed before midnight.

The most recent research shows that seven hours of sleep is the most ideal. So go to bed at eleven o'clock in the evening and wake up at six o'clock in the morning, which is the most ideal. Depending on the circumstances, it can vary, but try to stick to the most ideal.

Let us talk just a little bit about taking a nap, also known as siesta. There are some people who like to take a nap after lunch. There are some countries where napping is part of their culture. But first and most of all, you have to have a good night sleep and then take a nap. I do not recommend taking a nap after a bad night sleep. There is a distinct difference between napping and sleeping during the day. What I mean is napping is not daytime sleeping. If someone believes napping and daytime sleeping are the same, that person has to think again.

First and foremost, when you are napping, fifteen minutes are more than sufficient. If it is going over thirty minutes, it is no longer napping. It goes into the range of sleeping, i.e., daytime sleeping, which is hazardous to our body. I know someone who takes a nap every day after lunch for at least two hours. This is sleeping, not napping. What we need is napping, not sleeping.

Second, when we are napping, the depth of sleeping needs to go down to the first stage of sleeping. We do not need to go down to the second, third, or fourth stage of sleeping. When we are napping, we do not have to sleep. We just take a good rest with our eyes closed in a very comfortable posture for fifteen minutes or, at most, thirty minutes. Just close your eyes. That's all.

Proper napping will be an excellent medicine for our body, but daytime sleeping will be a poison to our body. Because we do not need the full four stages of sleep for napping. If we do, it will inter-fere our precious nighttime sleeping. What we need to achieve from napping is rest, not sleeping. All we need from a good napping is a good rest.

CHAPTER 12

How to Lose Weight: The One and Only and the Best

Losing weight? Are you sure? Yes, indeed. I have to give you something good in return for reading my book. If you are not convinced of my six elements of living healthy and long, at least you have something good to keep for the rest of your life hopefully. I'm telling you the best and the one and only way to lose weight. There is no other way. Only my way is the truth. But it is soon to be yours. It will be your truth and ours. I'm not saying that other people are lying when they are talking about weight loss. But they are not telling the truth, the whole truth. That's exactly what I mean. This is why.

Again, I'm writing this chapter in return for those people who spent their hard-earned money as well as their precious time reading this "boring" book of mine. I'm sure this book is very boring because my profession is not writing But some of you who have weight problem are going to have something in return, something called the "truth," my favorite word. For your precious time and money, I'm writing this chapter. I'm going to tell the truth for those who want to lose weight.

When you listen and stand with the truth, you might end up being alone but would never feel lonely because the truth is with you. I do not feel lonely when I'm alone with the truth. The truth that I'm about to tell you is not something that no one knows but is something that everyone knows already. If there is any truth that nobody knows, it is no longer truth. I'm putting the well-known truths together. When people, so-called experts, are focusing on one truth only, that's when they make this famous mistake. But the truth I'm about to tell you is the truth that everyone knows already. But if no one wants to tell you the truth the way it is and no one wants to look at this truth the way it is, then you are destined to fail. I'm going to help you face the truth exactly the way it is and overcome it and be successful. Who wants to come with me and be the winner?

I already told you that there are two kinds of truth—one that never changes and the other that changes with time.

Most of the truth does not change, and the fact does not change. Unfortunately, the truth that I'm about to discuss belongs to those that never change, no matter what. This truth will always be the same, so we are the ones who have to change, not the truth. The truth does not change. We have to change. Do not try to change or distort the truth. Then ultimately, we will be the ones who will suffer. The moment you look at the truth and make up your mind to face it, then you already achieved halfway of your goal. You are a half winner already. All you have to do is to take action, cross the finish line, and become a full and complete winner. The only small concern of mine regarding this truth, like any other truth, is that the road leading to this truth looks a bit narrower and seems a bit harder compared to the false truth, which always looks wide open, nicer, and easier. Too many people have wasted their precious time and enormous amount of money while pursuing the wrong truth and failed to achieve the goal. At the same time, so many elite physicians and scientists have devoted their valuable efforts to solve this problem and came up with an incomplete solution and failed. How many times have we heard a news that some scientists found the solution for obesity and then disappeared from our memory, like it never happened before?

Not too long ago, no sooner than Ms. Oprah Winfrey came out in a commercial and announced that she lost about twenty-eight pounds on a diet program of a certain diet company that not only the sales figure of that company went up sky-high but also its stock price. What a remarkable person she is. But no matter who the person might be, if you are not standing with the truth, there will be a time to crash and disappear from the horizon. The truth is we cannot solve an overweight issue with a diet program alone or exercise alone, to be honest.

How nice it would be if you can eliminate an overweight problem with one program. If someone tells you that they can eliminate an overweight issue with diet only or one pill only or exercise only, then that person is not telling you the truth. I did not say that person is lying.

Now here is the truth! I'm going to tell you the truth of gaining and losing weight at the same time. This is the truth of the cause of weight gain and weight loss, and as a result, it will lead you to the solution. You need to know both of the mechanisms of weight gain and loss simultaneously to achieve your goal, i.e., weight loss. If you know the cause of a problem, you are already halfway to solve the problem. Based on this truth, the cause and the solution for the weight gain and loss come simultaneously. It is the same thing with the moment you understand the cause of insomnia and you realize the answer at the same time. By the same token, the moment we understand the cause of weight gain, we know the answer. When you look at the truth the way it is, we are on the right track and at halfway of the finish line. You have to keep this in mind all the time while you are going through this simple truth. Because it is easy to remember and easy to forget. As they said, "Easy come, easy go." If you think losing weight is easy, you'll never lose weight.

Let's think that our body is a balloon. The more you blow a balloon, the bigger the balloon gets. The air goes in and does not come out. Where is the air that went inside? The simple answer is it stays inside.

Let's go back and think about the human body. When we eat food, ultimately the food will turn into calories that we use as our source of energy. But if we do not use the calories generated by the food, where do they go? Where do they stay? If ten people went inside and eight came out, where are the two? The truth is they are still inside. In the same way, the calories stay inside our body as a different form of energy source, such as glycogen in the muscle and the liver, as fats inside fat cells, and as fat cells itself under the skin of our belly, etc. Again, ten people went inside, and not only ten came out but also with two others. Altogether, twelve came out. What happened inside? There are two persons less inside. This is the truth, nothing but the truth, of weight loss. If someone says there is another way other than this, that person is not telling you the truth.

Now let's talk about the two truths of gaining weight—when and if you eat more than you spend and when and if you spend less than you eat. The remaining source of energy will remain in our body in the form of fat cells.

Let's face the other side of the truth, which is also the truth. Here come the two truths of losing weight—when and if we eat less than we spend and when and if we spend more than we eat. In order to make it easier to understand, I'm going to ask a question before we go any further. What is the best and the one and only way to spend (i.e., burn) energy (i.e., calories)? Many of you know the answer already. Yes, it is exercise. Exercise is the best way to kill and eliminate fat cells. There is no other way but to do exercise. Do you have any other way?

Again, this is how we gain weight—if we eat more than we exercise or if we exercise less than we eat. In other words, eat a lot and spend (exercise) less. Then you will gain weight.

Here comes the truth to lose weight—if we exercise more than we eat or if we eat less than we exercise. In other words, eat less and exercise more. Then you will lose weight. This is the best and one and only way to lose weight. There is no other way. So no matter how much more you eat, if you exercise more than you eat, you will lose weight. No matter how much less you eat, if you exercise less than you eat, you will gain weight.

As you can see, the solution based on the truth is exercise. But I'm not saying it is not important to watch what you are eating. It is very important what you are eating in terms of quality and quantity. For this, many of you already know better than I know. I'm emphasizing the importance of exercise, but that does not mean I'm ignoring the importance of what we are eating, i.e., diet.

There are many companies and people advertising their diet, their pill, their surgery, etc. No matter how good they might be, if we do not combine them with exercise, we are doomed to fail. That is the truth. If we do not exercise, we are going to fail. Plain and simple. If we do not incorporate exercise into our programs, our so-called effort will be wasted.

If we want to lose weight for whatever reason—such as diabetes, hypertension, hypercholesterolemia, or obesity itself, etc.—we have to focus on both ends, what you eat and how you exercise as well.

I agree that it is an excellent product that Marie Osmond is advertising. But if we choose to follow only her commercial's program or diet alone or anything without combining exercise, then we are destined to fail from the start or even before we start whatever we do.

So this is my way. Hopefully, it becomes yours too. Eat what you want, watch what you eat, and exercise! Remember exercise! You do not have to eat something that you do not like. Eat what you like but always remember something called "exercise."

I do not need to talk about diet or about what you eat in detail because you know already about these things better than I do. I do not need to talk about exercise in detail because you already read about the exercise in the chapter "Exercise, the Most Important of All."

Simply because it is difficult to face the truth, don't try to change or distort the truth. If you do that, the truth will become harder and cost you more financially, not to mention waste your valuable time.

I mentioned earlier that we have two kinds of truth—one that changes on its own and that has to be changed with time and one that never changes, no matter what happens.

Unfortunately, the truth of weight loss and sleeping belongs to the truth that never changes, no matter what. Because our body is made to be like that. Did we make our body to be like this? No, absolutely not!

Before we finish this chapter, let's do a simple math. The average calories we eat a day is about 2,200 kilocalories. If someone who is on average diet is burning 2,500 kilocalories a day, they will lose weight. But if the same person is burning only 2,000 kilocalories or less, they will gain weight. We cannot change this truth. And this is the result of the latest research that I agree 100 percent. It is kind of a new knowledge and very interesting. It is something that we should keep in mind about obesity, weight loss, etc.

I promised to discuss with you one thing before I finish this chapter. It is about the triple interrelationship among muscle cells, fat cells, and exercise.

It is possible to lose weight with diet only, but this research teaches us a valuable lesson that shows us how bad the result would be when we do it. It shows the ugly result of weight loss with diet only and without exercise. I'm going to explain it to you as if it happened to a real person.

Let's say, there was a healthy man, about forty years old. He, who liked to eat, started gaining weight. It has been known that when we are gaining weight, not only does the size of fat cells increase but also the number of fat cells. That's what happens around our belly, butt, neck, face, and everywhere in our body. Our belly looks like that of pregnant woman, our neck becomes two when there used to be one, and then our attractive double eyelid disappears one day without saying goodbye. One day, after shower, he looked at his body and was shocked at the way he looked in the mirror. He looked back and regretted what he had done so far. He realized that he ate too much steaks at dinner, cheeseburger at lunch, breakfast at Coney Island, snacks in between meals, like pizzas and chips with cola, etc. So he made up his mind to lose weight. He met with a well-known dietician and got a proven program. He followed the program. He was a very honest man and did not cheat. After six months, one year, and so on, he started losing weight. Finally, he succeeded to go back to his usual weight. He achieved his goal. And now he is looking at the truth in the mirror again.

The truth is the person he is looking at in the mirror is not the same person he once was. The one he used to be and the one in the mirror do not look the same and are actually different. He looks similar but not the same.

Let me explain. This is the truth scientists found, not I. When he gained his weight, as scientists said, the size and number of his fat cells increased. Hypothetically, when someone is losing weight with diet only and without exercise, from where does our body draw energy that we need? What is happening here? When we do not supply enough energy to our body, our body has to draw the necessary energy from inside our body. In these circumstances, our body has two major energy reservoirs—one is fat cells, and the other is muscle cells. So quite naturally, there will be two outcomes. One is when we lose weight with diet, our body attacks our muscle cells to draw energy to survive. So the majority of weight loss comes from muscle cells. The other is when we lose weight with exercise, our body attacks and kills fat cells to survive. Quite naturally, the majority of weight loss comes from fat cells. When someone loses weight with diet only and without exercise, the one in the mirror looks like the thumbnail of when one was overweight. Their belly is still out, the neck is still two, the butt is still out, etc. When someone loses weight with exercise, the one in the mirror looks like the one they used to be. The person will be so happy to see their previous self.

Who will be a happier person? I hope you are the happier person in real life after you lose your weight.

So the answer and the truth is when you want to lose weight, you have to exercise. At least you have to include and combine exercise in your program. If you do not include exercise in your program, it will inevitably fail from the beginning or even before the start, which I can guarantee.

To make it simple, the ideal weight loss is when you have to do it simultaneously: diet + exercise. Please do not do one alone. Combine the two. But if you want to lose weight with one method only, the answer is exercise. So the solution is exercise first, then combine it with diet or any program.

Always remember that exercise is the one that will get you to reach your goal. I hope you make a wise choice. Choose the truth.

CHAPTER 13

Isabella Stewart Gardner Museum

There is a big, or huge(?) museum in Detroit, Michigan, to be more exact, Dearborn, Michigan. By now, with location only, many people will recognize already which one I'm about to talk, even if you are not a resident of Detroit, or State of Michigan. Yes, it is Henry Ford Museum. Here, briefly, what I want to talk about is not the Henry Ford Museum, but much smaller one called Henry Ford Estate. It used to be a house, or mansion, or estate whatever you call at which Mr. Henry Ford lived until he fade away. I hate to use the word starting with d. Actually, he built this magnificent building for his one and only son, Edsel Ford (1893–1943) who died. No, fade away in his early forties. It is relatively small museum, but not many people living in Michigan know about this museum. It is located in Dearborn, the same city like Henry Ford museum and Greenfield Village. It takes only ten minutes or so drive by car.

When you get there and buy a ticket, a tour guide will meet you when the number of visitors reaches ten people or so.

When you go inside, the first thing(?) you will encounter is Model-T, with which Henry Ford (1863–1947) became billionaire or more than billionaire. It has been a while since my last visit. I only remember few things. To be honest, I remember three things.

First, visitors will meet three huge, industrial-size generators sitting next to each other. What? Generators? At a private home? But, not one, not two, three of them. Why three? Two are hydro, one is generator using coal. But, why three? This tells what kind of person who we are dealing with. One is not enough, if the first one is not working or goes out of order and stops, the entire mansion will go dark, pitch dark. Nothing will functioning. If one is not working, then the second one will do the work. While fixing number one, what if the second one goes out of order or stops. He has to have third one. What if the river runs dry due to drought, he has to have thermal generator using coal instead of hydro using water power.

Second, the house has a built-in vacuum cleaner. What? Vacuum cleaner? In the 1940s, did we have such thing? No way! But, he built a huge machine outside the house which is sucking out the air in the house. We can see a small hole, actually many holes on the floor. When needed, the house keeper put rubber hose into the hole, and turn on the switch and go after dusts, the machine sucks out the dust on the floor. And, collect the dust outside.

Third, the two old couple go out a picnic around noon with sandwiches and drinks in a basket. This activity becomes almost daily routine for them. But, they have to cross a creek, a branch of a river called River Rouge in front of the house. Then, the question is how. How did they cross the knee-high, or waist-high river when it rained the night before, Did they have a boat or a bridge built for the purpose of picnic? The answer is NO! Then, how? This is the answer. They built a dam away from the house for this particular purpose. When the time comes, he or she calls the housekeeper at the dam on the phone. Then, the person turns on the switch, and blocks the river. A stone bridge, or stepping stone will shows up to the surface. After crossing the river, one of the two calls again, the river goes back to original level. When they come back, same routine repeats.

There is a museum in Boston named Isabella Stewart Gardner Museum, also known as Fenway Court, in the middle of the city. The museum has lots of valuable and famous artworks. I recommend very highly that many of you should visit this museum and see an artwork or more—not to see the artworks which are not there. I'm telling you the conclusion first, which is you are paying money to see some artworks which are not there anymore, to be exact, which were stolen in 1990, twenty-seven-some years ago.

There are not many people who remember this event now. Even the people living in Boston do not know and remember about this any longer. Just looking at the name, it sounds like a Spanish queen's name, but her father originally came from Ireland and her mother from England. Both of her parents were born in very rich families. In those days, majority of immigrants were poor or very poor, but her parents were one of the few exceptions.

Isabella Stewart was born in 1840 in upper class New York. She was the oldest of four siblings, but the younger ones died in their young ages that she became the only one who inherited all her parents' fortune. She did not attend a public school or private school. Excellent teachers came to her house.

Between the ages of sixteen and eighteen, she went to Paris for better education along with her parents, which tells how rich they were.

After she came back from Europe, she met her future husband, Jack Gardner, when she was visiting her friend who also went to Paris for the same reason with her brother, and they became friends. They got married in April of 1860. They had a son who died of pneumonia at the age of two. It was not uncommon that not only babies but also even adults died due to pneumonia because penicillin was yet to be invented. No matter how rich they might be, they could not buy penicillin. Simply, it was yet to be invented.

Quite naturally, the rich couple made a desperate effort to have another child. But each time she got pregnant, the pregnancy ended up with natural abortion, also known as habitual abortion, which means her female organ could not sustain the fetus through full term. Based on nineteenth-century medical science, they had no choice but to give up having another child. When she was told there's no choice, she fell into a severe depression. With the doctor's advice, the couple decided to travel the world.

At that time, commercial airline was not yet available, but they visited almost everywhere in the world. Of course, their favorite countries are Europe, Africa, Asia, etc. Of course, they visited Egypt and countries like Japan, Thailand, and so on. That was how she was able to overcome her depression, by traveling.

The couple moved to Boston and began their lives devoting and contributing deeply to the city of Boston, including art collection. One of the local reporters wrote, "Mrs. Jack Gardner is one of the seven wonders of Boston. There is nobody like her in any city in this country."

In 1884, she traveled to Japan again, China, Cambodia, and Egypt as well. She also visited England, and her interest and knowledge in art and art collection got deeper and deeper. In 1891, her father passed away, and she inherited all her parents' fortune. In 1898, her husband died suddenly of stroke. Since the death of her husband, she began to build a museum called Fenway Court and displayed all her collections while living on the top floor of the museum. She developed and maintained a relationship with artists and art collectors in Europe and put much more efforts in art collection.

In December 1919, she herself became hemiplegic after a stroke and died in July 1924. Before she died, she donated everything she owned to the city of Boston with one condition, which is to keep everything exactly the way she displayed. She did not want to look any of her art collection moved or changed or different from what she had done in Fenway Court, which was her baby. But in March of 1990, ninety-five years after she died, there was an "accident" that broke her wishes completely. It was in March in Boston, and it was still cold. Especially in the midnight of March.

Ever since the museum changed the name from Fenway Court to Isabella Stewart Gardner Museum, it would open at eight o'clock in the morning and close at five o'clock in the afternoon, and all the employees would go home, including the director of the museum, except for two security guards who would stay until the next morning. At five o'clock in the afternoon, when everybody would have gone home, the security guards would shut all the museum's doors and would not open the doors until the next morning, no matter what the reason might be. If somebody, including the director, forgot something, then the person who forgot something could complete the unfinished business the next day, although only the director had the authority to open the door after hours.

However, while even the director was not aware of what was going on, something truly unthinkable happened on that night. CNN had a one-hour special report about this art theft three to four years ago, which I'm going to recall as much as I can.

It was around midnight of March 18, 1990. It was about time when—as a routine, one of the two security guards was making rounds while the other one was sitting on the front desk, monitoring the entire facility—the doorbell on the rear entrance rang.

Think about what is available now and what was not available over twenty-five years ago. In terms of security system of the twenty-first century of now and the twentieth century of then, there is a tremendous difference. Some equipment which are everywhere and available now, such as CCTV (closed-circuit television) or GPS and so on, were still yet to be seen. We can only see the walkie-talkie they were using for communication between two persons at children's toy stores, such as Toys "R" Us.

By the way, motion detector was available then. So when the security guard at the control center looked at the monitoring screen, he saw two uniformed Boston police officers at the rear door, asking or "demanding" to open the door. Instead of saying no, the security guard asked why they needed to get in. One of the disguised thieves yelled back that there was an urgent call from inside the museum reporting a significant disturbance and that they had to get in and investigate what was going on. The security guard in the control center went into panic mode. All of a sudden, in the middle of the night, like in *Hamlet*, he asked himself, "To be or not to be?" This poor man was stuck between the two questions, "To open?" or "Not to open?" Actually, he went into panic, only thinking, "Should I open or not?" But out of the confusion, without having a chance to discuss about the matter with his partner, he went into panic deeper and deeper.

Even though he had other two choices to get out of the situation easily, his brain stopped functioning only to the question of "To open or not to open?" Apparently, he had two choices which were very easy. Both of the two were just one phone call away. One was to call his director at home, who would be in bed sleeping with his phone next to his bed, and then asked just one question, "Should

I open the door?" And the other one was to call the precinct with which the museum had a direct phone line. He could ask just one question, "Did you send two officers to us?"

When they came inside, they were pretending to look for something or anything unusual while asking several questions to the security guard. Then suddenly, one of the fake policemen yelled at the security guard, saying, "You look exactly like the murder suspect! The picture of you was posted on the wall today!" Then he pulled out his gun and ordered the security guard to go to the wall and turn around and face the wall. As soon as the security guard stood facing the wall, his hand was put on a handcuff instantaneously.

By then, the other security guard came down from the second floor. The moment he asked what was going on to his partner, he was also handcuffed at gunpoint. They were taken down to the boiler room in the basement and locked up until they were found by their employee the next day after a long search. Because their mouths were duct-taped, they could not talk to each other or scream for help to release them or explain what happened.

According to the motion detector, it happened around midnight. There was no movement whatsoever until two o'clock in the morning, and then the action began. The thieves waited for two hours without doing anything while making sure everything was on the right track as planned. And they disappeared around five o'clock in the morning. They took thirteen items, of which the total worth was estimated to be five hundred millions. Among the stolen items, *The Concert*, which is one of Vermeer's paintings, is being estimated to be over two hundred million alone. Although I do admit that I'm not an expert in art, I value more the painting by Rembrandt, *The Storm on the Sea of Galilee*.

But why only thirteen items? For two hours, they occupied the entire museum. Why only thirteen? This is one of the puzzles that the FBI special units could not solve or explain why until now. First of all, there were more valuable artworks than those two, but they did not take more valuables. Why? And why only thirteen? Why not more? They had sufficient time to take more than that.

If you go to the Dutch Room on the second floor, you are going to see the wall where the two famous paintings were hanging has two gigantic frames hanging without paintings inside. They took those two paintings down on the floor, cut them out with razor-sharp knife, rolled the paintings, put the paintings inside a paper cylinder, and then took them. You know the reason why they did not take as many as they could. Actually, no one knows why, but you know the rest of the story.

So when you go into the Dutch Room and if you look at the wall carefully just above the fireplace, you will notice the two giant frames without paintings inside hanging on the wall. If you stand in front of the wall, all you will see is the wall. Where you are supposed to see the paintings, you won't see any. You will only see the wall. If you turn around and see the opposite side, you will see the self-portrait of young Rembrandt looking at you, or the wall, where one of his masterpieces was proudly hanging.

But ironically, no one seems to pay attention to this empty exhibition, even though lots of people—young and old and male and female—are coming in and then going out, without questioning why the wall is empty. Certainly, I could not find any notice explaining what happened or why the wall has frames only, without paintings. Although Rembrandt himself—to be exact, his self-portrait—must have seen exactly what happed on that night, he is silent. He does not say anything, although he saw everything.

I became a bit upset while watching the empty wall that I started talking to myself, which only I could hear, "Who did this? Who are these SOBs? What a genius he is? What is his IQ?"

And there was a group of people who seemed to be having a field trip filled with laughing and giggling to one another. So I talked to the lady who seemed to be the leader of the group. "Do you know the reason why the frames on the wall do not have paintings?"

She said, "Oh, no." Then immediately, she added, "What? Did you say the paintings on the wall do not have paintings? What do you mean by that?"

I told her that I could explain the reason why exactly if she gave me an opportunity to tell the entire group, who was about twenty people altogether. So I spent five to ten minutes of time to explain everything. When I finished, everybody said all at the same time, "Oh my god!"

Yes, indeed, it's "Oh my god!" This is a tragedy to all of us. It is a tragedy not only for those who did it but also for those of us who cannot see it with our very own eyes.

Please help us, God. Move those hearts who did it to turn in those artworks to the lawful and rightful owner, the museum, and all of us.

After twenty-seven years, it is about time for those who planned the thief and succeeded to do something right this time. Return them. You may not be able to return those artworks through the rear entrance door where you came in on that night because it is not existing anymore. It was demolished. You can return them through the front door. Or if you think it is too much for you to return them through the front door, then you have a much easier way to do the right thing at last. Return them to me. I can and will return them to the rightful owner for you. If you read my book, you know who I am. I'm more than willing to do the heavy lifting for you. You took them for free. You should return them for free. I'll make you free, whether you are the one who took them or who owns them. Do not feel sorry when you return them because you took them without paying, not even with a single penny. They belong to the museum and ultimately to all of us. Let all of us, all the humanity, enjoy the magnificent creations of one of our own humanity. Do not take away the privilege from us and only enjoy it with just a few of you or only you. I guarantee you that you will be a much happier person when you see all our faces turn so happy. I definitely do not think your goal is money. I think you achieved your goal already on that faithful night. Simply you can send them to me. I'll return the treasures as soon as I receive them to the rightful owner, the museum, and ultimately the people. I'll be waiting and waiting from the moment my book is published. You know me. I'm giving you the best chance to make up your behavior. You know who I am if you read this book.

Alaska

You can travel Alaska in a group or with a few. For example, you can do it in a group with your families, such as on a wedding anniversary, seventieth birthday, etc. You can do it with a few. In my case, it was two couples—me and my wife and my best friend and his wife—also known as Special Force of Travel Unit, like the Navy SEALs of a travel agency. Set the goal, research and study, attack the enemy, and return home safe.

I do not mind which one you choose, depending on your situation, but I recommend my way, with which you will get a better result in terms of a spiritual or soulful journey. Always remember that if you travel in a group, always there is one or two rotten apples in the basket.

The history of Alaska is rather short but a bit interesting. When you are watching a professional sports game on TV and when the team you are rooting for is winning the game, the game becomes more interesting. When the Russian Empire and the premature stage of America were involved in a political game on the issue of Alaska, it appeared that Russia was on the winning side in the beginning. At the time of the signing ceremony, at least Russia was thinking definitely it was on the winning side. Because when the representatives of Russia and America went back their own countries, they received the exact opposite reception from their countries. Guess who received the enthusiastic and who received the chilling reception?

The representative of America received the most chilling response you will ever think of. Because he was blamed for purchasing a land with a weather of winter cold for the entire year and frozen most of the year that it could not grow anything from the ground, could not raise farm animals, and was filled with dangerous animals.

In Moscow, meanwhile, there was a huge party celebrating the huge success. They were whispering to one another's ears, "Those big-nosed Yankees have no brains" for buying a wasteland with such a huge money.

In Washington, there was a motion to fire the secretary of the state in Congress for making such a lousy deal with Russia with an enormously high price. As you can tell, Alaska belonged to Russia, until the time of the destiny, which was March 30, 1867, when the treaty was signed.

Quite naturally, in those days, quite a lot of Russians, not Americans, were living in Alaska. And as a matter of fact, Russia needed Alaska to make fur coats, fur hats, and so on. The fur coats and fur hats that Dr. Zhivago and Sasha were wearing in the movie *Doctor Zhivago* might have come from Alaska and might have been made from Alaskan furry animals. To catch furry animals, the Russians even came down to northern California. The Russians desperately needed animal furs to make fur coats, jackets, mittens, and hats to warm up their bodies. We all saw the movie *Doctor Zhivago*.

Initially, the Russians themselves went out to the wild and caught the furry animals. But the job was not easy for the Russians. To them, the Alaskan people, i.e., the Eskimos, were far better hunters and had far better skills than them. Instead of venturing into the Alaskan wilderness risking their lives, they began to buy the furry animals' skins captured by the Alaskans with a certain amount of money, which must have been very cheap. But the money was too precious that they did not want to pay for the furry animals. So they asked the Russian government to send the troops to Alaska to take the furs away from the Eskimos at gunpoint. If the Eskimos refused to go out and catch the animals, the troops would take one of the families as hostage and release the hostage if the young Eskimos bring enough furs. Such an atrocity ended when the Russians sold Alaska to America and signed the treaty.

If you go around Alaska, occasionally you will be able to see a small or large cemetery of the Russians who lived in the area in the past. What kind of an irony is that that when you died, you were buried in your country, and then all of a sudden, you are buried in somebody else's land? Probably, what will the Russians—especially the leaders of the country, for example, Mr. Putin—think whenever they see Alaska on the map that belongs to America since 1867 and realize that, before 1867, it was the land of Russia?

Do you know how big Alaska is? It is 1,717,856 square kilometers, i.e., 663,268 square miles. If compared to Korea, North and South combined, it is 219,155 square kilometers bigger. It is eight times the size of the entire Korean Peninsula. Just imagine it is almost ten times of Korea, again North and South combined. It is bigger than Texas and also bigger than California. It's the biggest state of the United States of America. For that, Russia received 7.8 million dollars, which means $0.02 per acre or $4.74 per square meter. It was a huge amount of money at that time, but let's think about the current value of Alaska.

Can you imagine the current economic value of Alaska in dollars? And then the geopolitical value? Can you describe the strategic value in dollars? What about the strategic and the military value of Alaska? What about its value for the security of Canada and USA? Have you ever thought about the value of Alaska, combining all the above?

We can make a simple formula, which is very simple, whether it is especially and strategically something good for America but bad for Russia or something bad for America but good for Russia.

But no matter how good or bad the deal was then and is now, if you do not go and put your feet on the land and move around Alaska, you will never realize how good and how bad it is to whom. And another important thing we have to keep in mind is that no matter how good and how bad the deal was and is, we cannot change the deal once it was signed by both. That is the reason why you have to think twice—no, more than a dozen times—when you sign a contract, not only when it is a personal contract but, more importantly, when it is between two countries. You cannot turn back time. You cannot announce the contract is illegal.

Let's go back to traveling. We had enough talk about international politics. Back to Alaska!

I mentioned before that it is better with a few of your very close friends for traveling Alaska. It was very helpful that my friend's wife had been to Alaska several times in the past because her close relatives were living in Fairbanks, Alaska.

Big cruise ships depart from Seattle or Vancouver, Canada, and then sail north along the coastline. I heard the cruise ships provide very excellent entertainment program. But I hope all of you who traveled Alaska already and who are planning to travel Alaska in the near future have some kind of spiritual journey or a similar kind while or after the Alaska visit.

This happened to be my "spiritual" experience. I hope all of you to have the same experience like I had. Yes, this is my way, and this is my opinion. Somebody can have a different idea.

As I said more than once in this book, timing is important. My window period of traveling Alaska is approximately from early July to late August. I'd like to go to Alaska in the winter. But I'd like to go twice in the summer rather than once in wintertime. Unless you have to, I would not go to Alaska in June or before July or in September or after August, which means I would go to Alaska only in July or August.

Take an airplane and go to Anchorage, Alaska. Those people living in Canada or in the northern states in the US go to Alaska with their own RV (recreational vehicle) or rented RV. It may take between seven to eight hours of flight from Seoul, South Korea, to Anchorage, Alaska. At the airport, you can rent a car that fits your own itinerary and your personality. It can be a four-door sedan, an SUV, a minivan, or an RV. Unlike other airports, you can rent an RV in the Anchorage airport. Then you can go wherever you want to go. You can use GPS if you need direction. You need to look at the map once in a while. For direction, you listen to the Google GPS lady, instead of using the map.

So from Anchorage, you go north in a very early morning and arrive at a coastal town, Weawold, where you hop on a ship to tour the glacier. It takes eight hours for a round trip of sightseeing. The ship will stop by more than several places that you will remember long after your trip to Alaska. One of the sightseeing that you will remember is watching the humpback whales right in front of your own eyes. What a sight!

Then to the glacier! You will watch the glacier from the sea. I described to the best of my ability the glacier in the Canadian Rocky Mountains, where I was standing on the top of the glacier.

As you know, I'm not a man of books, neither of reading or writing. I honestly confess to all of you that it is impossible for me to write or describe many things that I'm writing in this book. This is one of the many. Glacier! Glacier! Glacier! That's all I can do. Instead of describing it, I have to dare to ask you questions that I can think of. First, "Glacier, glacier, how old are you?" Second, "Where did you get the color you have? Where did you get the wonderful color?" Third, "How do you make that sound? What is the secret of the amazing sound you are making when you are falling into the sea? Where did you get that voice? How do your vocal cord and voice box look like?" Fourth, "Why are you falling down at this moment? Why now? Why are you trying to come close to me? How long did you wait for me? Why me? Who are you? And who am I?"

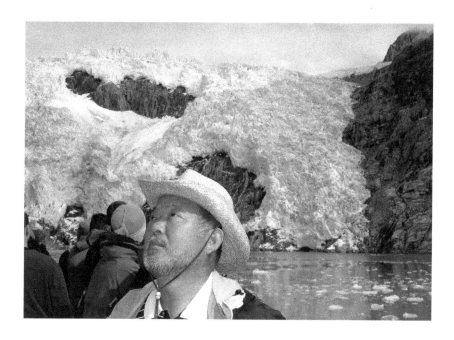

All I can tell you is this is the performance of nature, created by someone upstairs. But among the performances, the most memorable and amazing moment is not the visual; it is the audio. This way, I do not have to describe the glacier, and I am leaving it up to you and your imagination. Now it is up to you. You have to go like me. Seeing is believing it. But this is one of the many moments of supernatural, spiritual, soulful experiences while traveling.

The only thing I feel sorry about the glacier is it is shrinking. It is going on even now and getting faster and faster because of global warming. There are many people, especially among the many leaders of major political parties and major religious groups, who do not believe and even deny what they are looking at. What kind of hypocrite are they? Where did they come from? Other planets? I have no problem accepting the difference of opinions, none whatsoever! But this one is a fact. Why do many people say nothing is happening when clearly something is happening right in front of their own eyes? Where are they from? Or do they know or see something I do not know or see? If so, please share with us what you know or see.

The next day, in the early morning, we headed to Denali, the second tallest mountain in the world other than the Himalaya. It has been called Mount McKinley, named after William McKinley who was born and raised in Ohio; became the twenty-fifth president of the US; was assassinated in 1901, six months into the second term; and has nothing to do with Alaska. Among the Alaskan Indians, it has been called Mount Denali, which means tall and high mountains. From a distance, the native Indians would show their respect to it and call it the tall one. They wanted this tall one to have its own name, the Denali. It was their dream to call the tall one "tall." Finally, last year in the summer of 2016, President Obama went to the park—a few years before, I stood and took pictures of my traveling partners and me with Denali behind—and had an official ceremony to call it Denali, officially for good, no more Mount McKinley. Mr. Obama did a very good thing to native Americans and the tall one, Denali. Dream did come true for the native American Indians.

Here is something about American Indians and Koreans. Both of these two people originated from the same place—meaning, they had the same ancestors. A long, long time ago, probably thousands of years ago, they originated from the Ural and Altai mountains in Central and East Asia—where Russia, China, Mongolia, and Kazakhstan come together—and migrated through upper China and Southern Russia and then separated in Manchuria. Majority of the group came down to and settled in the Korean Peninsula, and some continued and crossed the sea and went to Japan islands. The other group continued, crossed the Bering Strait, moved to the American continent, and became the native American Indians. If you look at any American Indian and me standing next to each other, you will find many undeniable similarities between us.

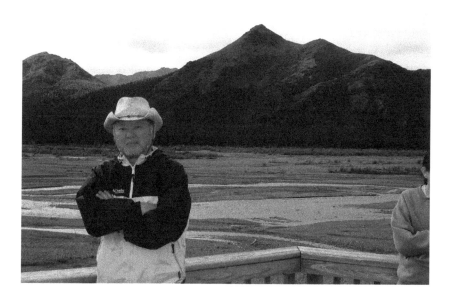

Before arrival to the Denali National Park, there is a small park with a viewing area, where we stood and look at Denali and took pictures of it. A few years later after me, Mr. Obama came and look at Denali and took pictures where we took pictures. Among the tall mountains, with white snows on the top in the middle of the summer and thick clouds around the shoulder, there it is, the tallest one among the tall ones, being called by the natives and now by all Americans Denali.

Again, wake up in the early morning and go to the Denali National Park. Inside the park office, we found out that we could not go any farther with our car. The parking lot is the finish line. You have to take the park bus to go inside. There are many options—half-day or full-day tour. And another option is if you are a hiker, the bus will drop you off at a certain place, where you can camp or spend the night at a cottage, and then pick you up the next day at the same time and place.

You can plan ahead what to do at Denali National Park if you go on the website. We took the eight hours' tour with other tourists in a bus. The bus driver was also the tour guide. We had no idea how deep and how high we were going inside. But just imagine it was four hours of one-way trip. And sometimes the bus ran pretty fast in flat plains, and other times, it slowed down when it went on pretty dangerous steep hills. On the way and back, if you are lucky, you will see wild animals. We all know that we can see those animals at the nearby zoo, but it's an entirely different feeling if you see those animals in the wild. You can see a deer or moose and sometimes elks and caribous when you drive in the remote mountainous area, if you are lucky. The elks or caribous especially did not run away when we approached, although the deer ran away as soon as we made eye-to-eye contact. So when you see an elk or caribou, you can approach as close as you can and exchange conversation nonverbally.

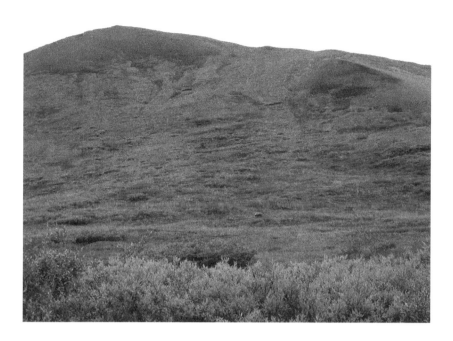

We saw bears on two separate occasions, one as a family and the other as a lone adult bear. The park bus driver, also the tour guide, suddenly stopped the bus and told us to look at a certain area of a creek in a distance. A family of four—one mama bear and three baby bears—crossed the creek and then disappeared into the woods. The second encounter was we were a bit lucky. Suddenly, the bus slowed down and stopped. The bus driver whispered to us to look to the right side of the bus. There he was! An adult bear was almost next to us, sitting in the bushes and picking up and eating mountain berries with his hands. He was so focused on minding his business that he did not care that the bus stopped right next to him or not. He continued what he was doing. Then he stood up and walked slowly to the opposite direction from us and disappeared. What an experience! It's like a close encounter of the third kind in the wild. All of us had to say goodbye to his huge butt.

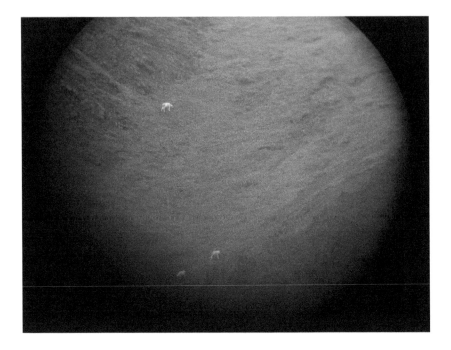

Here's another lucky encounter of wild animals. This time, it was mountain goats, when the bus stopped for a break at a place with a few small cottagelike buildings and outside bathrooms. Not very far from us, we could see a rolling river too. We were walking around and talking to one another about how lucky we were and so on. Somehow, there were four or five binoculars standing outside, the kind we can see in any metro or national parks that we paid not much attention. Again, the bus driver and tour guide as well told us to look at the mountain slopes close to the top carefully and see if we can find multiple white spots slowly moving. Indeed, there were many white spots in a group of almost fifteen to twenty moving slowly in one direction. When we told him what we were seeing, he told us to look at them with the binoculars next to us. Now we could tell what those white spots were. We could tell the heads, trunks, and legs. Yes, they were moving slowly, but they were doing something while moving. They were eating. They were eating grasses while moving. That's why they were slow. But to me, although with the help of binoculars, I could not see any grasses.

Suddenly, something came to my mind out of nowhere. I asked the tour guide a very interesting question. "Why are they staying up there in the first place? To me, I cannot see any grasses up so high. I see only rocks, no grasses or trees up there. Through the binocular, I saw only rocks where they were in all different sizes and shapes. If they come down here, I see a bunch of green grasses all around us. And a lot of water too."

My tour guide kindly explained to me and the others the reason why. "It is some kind of survival of the fittest. When and if they come down, it will be extremely lucky for them to have lots and lots of grasses everywhere. A lot of food and water as well. But there is one catch here. It would be always good to have enough food around them, but they can be excellent food for another hungry animal down here, mainly wolves, the predators of the mountain goats. Yes, on rare occasions, they do come down here because they were too hungry or too stupid. Sometimes we see the leftovers. Of course, some of the wolves who are too hungry or too smart go up the mountain to hunt for food. But usually, they are unsuccessful. Most of the time, they come back with empty hands, certainly empty stomachs. Because on the ground level, the wolves run fast, certainly faster than the goats. It's no match. But up in the mountain with a rocky surface, the goats are faster than the wolves. Because their feet are well adjusted to that particular harsh environment. You know that the goats are excellent rock climbers, don't you?"

Indeed, it is survival of the fittest.

When we were done with the Denali tour, the sun was about to go down. We had to find a place to have a nice dinner and a decent hotel or motel. We found a good restaurant and had a nice dinner, but we got even luckier that we found an excellent motel, as it turned out to be later. We were driving to the direction of Fairbanks, our next destination. In the middle of nowhere, we found one with "vacancy" light on. We went inside the office and asked for two rooms and then went into the room. We found out that the room was a passenger compartment of a retired, old-fashioned train. They had done such an excellent job in insulation that once we turned on the heater, it turned into a warm and cozy and very much romantic place. I was able to hear the wind blowing, the trees shivering, the small animals playing with each other under my room, and the cry of wolves from a distance, and so on. When the sun went down and the darkness fell on us, though we were the ones thrown into the Alaskan wilderness, I did not feel isolated or lonely at all. I felt like I was sleeping in my bed.

Then we stopped by Fairbanks, drove to the north, and arrived at a small town, Chene. It was too small that there were only a few traffic signals in it. But I saw a small airport close to the town for the wealthy people with the private jets coming from everywhere, even from New York, etc. Why? For what? Because this town has hot springs. It is outdoor. It is so hot that you can see the steam going up from the hot spring. You cannot stay a while near the hot water springs. You have to keep some distance. If you go to the hot spring after dinner or after dark, you can see all the stars in the sky, the Alaskan sky. I felt like the stars twinkled right in front of my nose. It was so romantic!

CHAPTER 15

Dental Hygiene

Gum disease and halitosis. First of all, this is not my area of expertise, so I have to be careful when I talk about someone else's issues. Even if I make a wrong statement, please be kind and generous because it is totally unintentional. These two headaches are extremely important issues. But by just talking about these, I might hurt the feelings of the good people from the dental department without achieving my goal. So I put this chapter almost at the end of my book.

It is absolutely absurd that I'm talking about this because there are so many experts, also known as dentists, around us who spent the golden years of their lives studying this science. But dentists are reluctant to tell their patients who have this problem, especially halitosis, which is their responsibility to discuss and treat. But once you talk about this, there is a high chance to lose your patients. So they choose not to talk about this rather than lose their valuable patients.

So somebody has to speak up. And that somebody happens to be me, who does not know too much about this important problem of ours. Who will be the one to put the alarm bell on the neck of a cat—oh no, on the neck of a tiger or lion? Am I crazy? But if not me, who is going to be the one?

In fact, I had this problem also and lived with it for a long, long time until recently I found the solution. The solution that I found happens to be so good that I want to share this with more people. Actually, there are many people already who are practicing it every day with excellent outcome. As you know already, when I discuss about health issues, I always put the answer, i.e., the solution, at the end of the chapter. And the solutions are not my own creation or something that nobody knows. I am not the one who created or found the answer. In fact, those solutions are someone else's, not mine. None of those is mine. The only thing I did is put them together. That's all. Actually, like the others, the solutions that I recommend are already known to most of the people. So the solution of gum disease and halitosis is well-known to the public. It is not my own creation.

When I talk to people about these issues, approximately two out of ten are using my method already. This chapter is dedicated to those eight out of ten people who know about this magic but are not taking advantage of it. I also learn this magic from one of my patients, and I shared this magic with my other patients and friends before, and then I am sharing this magic with you now. If you are one of the eight out of ten, I hope you find this magic like I did and keep it for the rest of your life. By the way, I forgot the name and the face of the patient who passed his torch to me. But I hope I do the same to you the way he did. You can forget me. I give you the permission to forget me, but I hope you do not forget what I'm about tell you in this chapter.

Let me ask you a question before I talk about dental hygiene. Some of you know the answer already. What are the three dirtiest parts of our body? I'll give you the three. Try to rank them from the worst, but put the worst on the top. This list is random:

* the opening at the end of the gastrointestinal tract
* the two openings—one on the right and one on the left—on the face just behind both eyes called ear canals or, to be exact, the external ear canals
* the mouth—actually, inside the mouth—which we are about discuss

Depending on how you manage them, the ranking could be different. But the worst are the ear canals. The next is our mouth.

Then the cleanest of the three is the opening at the end of the gas-trointestinal tract.

Why are ear canals the worst? The only way we can clean this area is with Q-tips, but without seeing it. How do we know we are actually cleaning when we think we are cleaning? Thought and reality do not necessarily go hand in hand all the time. Have you ever heard of perforating the eardrums when we are cleaning our ear canals by pushing the Q-tips a bit too deeper and then losing the ability of hearing later? I have seen and witnessed so many victims of Q-tips. Even with Q-tips, how do you know you cleaned well? Did you see it? Have you seen your ear canals with your own eyes ever in your life?

Next is the mouth. We brush our teeth every day. But brushing the teeth does not necessarily mean cleaning the teeth or mouth. The mission is not yet accomplished. The explanation comes soon.

Next is the opening at the end of our gastrointestinal tract, also known as anus. Many people take a shower every day, like we brush our teeth every day. We clean this area so good because we think this area is the dirtiest area of our body. So we make sure this area is real clean, and we do it so obsessively that we do not even have to look at it because we are sure it is clean. Is there anyone who checks their rear end on the mirror to see if it was cleaned thoroughly? I do not. Actually, no one does. We don't need to. Because we know we cleaned this area real good when we use our hand and fingertip on this most sensitive part of our body.

However, we are going to start the mission to make our mouth the cleanest part of our body. I do not have to explain that if we main-tain our oral hygiene well or not, not only our quality of life but also our financial aspect would be drastically different. There is a saying, "Good teeth, long life." This is not because we have a government-is-sued statistics or a result of research from a big university's dental department. It is the wisdom of life that comes from our elderly, handed from generation to generation. However, it is those people with serious dental problem who do not believe this generational wisdom more than those with decent dental hygiene, those with little or no problem with their teeth. Simply speaking, it is just a matter of time that someone who has bad teeth would mess up their stomach because their bad mouth, due to poor dental hygiene, cannot chew or grind the food properly and does not give well-mixed food that is ready for digestion to the stomach. This means that dental health and the stomach have the same destiny; as the dental hygiene goes down, the stomach is destined to go down. They go down together. I do not know too much about Buddhism, but Buddha taught, "Life is the ocean of pain," which means our lives are filled with pain and hardship that we have to deal with. But despite the pain and hardship, there is pleasure, and one of the rare pleasures in our lives is the pleasure of food and the pleasure of eating the food we like.

Whenever we eat, we eat for the pleasure only, not to mention for the preservation of species. So to increase and extend our pleasure is by eating slow and longer. I'm the happiest man on earth when I put a certain food that I like the most into my mouth. If someone is envious about what I just said, I'll give you the answer to get rid of your envy right away. I'm going to give you exactly how to get rid of gum disease in your mouth. How nice it would be if you do not have this evil.

When you get rid of gum disease with my recommendation, there is another evil one that disappears from your mouth. That evil one is called halitosis. One evil goes away. Wow! One more and the two evils go away from your mouth as evil as or eviler than the first one. Wow!

Causing symptoms of psychiatric illnesses, the mind is so unstable that the patient sees something that is not there, hears voices or noises which are not there, and feels even though nobody or nothing is touching them. We call this unusual phenomenon hallucination, which could be visual, auditory, and tactile. Does this mean that the foul odor coming out of our mouth is so bad that we can have a hallucination? Is that why we gave it the same first name? "Hal—"? In Chinese language, they call the bad-mouth smell, i.e., halitosis, "evil smell." At this point, I'm going to leave it up to your imagination how bad it is literally. It is up to your interpretation, but it tells the problem that we are talking about is very serious.

Anyway, it is not that easy to explain the definition of halitosis itself, but it is much more difficult to talk to people because there is a vast area of misunderstanding about this problem. In other word, it is easy to hurt someone's feeling, the pride of someone. This is so much a sensitive issue that I would not recommend to discuss or comment about this, no matter how close you are among your families or your friends. Just leave it up to them until they find out the solution their own way. And be patient because it is too personal. Leave this sensitive and difficult issue to a person like me or a book like this one.

Halitosis is the by product or end product of two evils   inflam mation of the gums and decomposing foods stuck in between the teeth, which will not only damage our health with the smell itself but also will give us bad influence in our interpersonal relationship. For example, just imagine that whenever a leading man, like Clark Gable or Leonardo DiCaprio, opens his mouth and bad smell comes out, what would happen to the leading lady who has to talk in a very close distance and has to kiss him many times throughout the moviemaking? Or what if a physician, an internist, who has to perform a physical examination all day extremely close to their patients has bad smell coming from their mouth? Or what if a genius who just graduated from Harvard or MIT (Massachusetts Institute of Technology) and is recently hired by a high-tech company talks to the company's CEO in close range about a very important future project or vice versa? The more important the project is, the closer the distance between the two will be. Or what if a young man who is in love with the girl of his dream is about to kiss her and his bad smell comes out of his mouth with a nicotine flavor?

However, there is something we have to pay attention to, something we have to keep in mind. The person who has this problem does not know of the fact that they have the problem. My explanation for this phenomenon is we have a body that has a superexcellent ability to adjust to any environment we are under, whether good or bad, easy or difficult, small or big, etc. In this case, the olfactory nerve inside our nose has an excellent ability to adjust to this environment by quitting its function or numbing itself instantaneously. No matter how bad or good the smell might be, if it is too strong, we do not smell it the way it is after a few seconds. For example, we smell the strong fragrance of roses, but within a few seconds, we do not smell it as strong as it is. This is why some or many are living with this problem for a long, long time or all their lives without recognizing it. If someone knows that they have this problem, then the person is doing something or anything already and may be successful already.

This is a true story. In the past, in China, there was a national hero whose name was Mao Tse Tung. As the leader in his Communist party, he unified China, which became the largest and biggest nation in the history of all China. There was no emperor, king, or general who achieved and unified China as Mao did. There was no one like Mao in China's history, no one before and no one after.

When he became the chairman of the Communist party, a dentist was assigned to him and his family. Later on, the dentist requested for a political asylum to the US government and lived somewhere in the US until he died. He wrote his autobiography. In his autobiography, he wrote a story of a person who had a really bad smell from his mouth. That person's name is Mao, the chairman. It was probably because he was too busy. If it's for that reason, I fully understand. But in reality, not only he had never come to his dentist, who only treated his family, but also never brushed his teeth in his entire life. No matter how his personal dentist might have threatened him, he had never come and seen his dentist. So as you can imagine, his "fragrance" followed him wherever he went and whenever he saw his fellow citizens or foreign dignitaries. Once, he told his concerned dentist, pointing to the big Siberian tiger in the picture hanging on a giant wall, "Have you ever seen any tiger seeing the dentist?" But there is something funny that you have to keep in mind. If any tiger overheard about this conversation, the tiger might say, "Even as tigers, we, living in the twenty-first century, also see our dentist during our annual checkup, like any people."

Even though we humans have a very excellent smell system as sensitive as any other animals, we are very generous to the smell coming from ourselves, which means no matter how bad our smell might be, it does not make us feel uncomfortable. But it makes us very uncomfortable if the bad smell comes from others. Because of this rule of nature, a similar smell from me does not bother me, but if it comes from others, it bothers me. This strange phenomenon occurs to couples too. When your bad smell and your partner's bad smell mix together and become your smell, it does not bother both of you anymore. That is the reason why you live your lives happily ever after.

When I was little, most of my "fellow citizens" lost their teeth because of decay. We did not have good toothbrushes and toothpaste like we have now. We did not have fluoride in the drinking water either. So in the past, when we lost our tooth, the tooth looked ugly and dirty with part of it missing.

Now we do not lose our tooth because of decay anymore. Now we lose our tooth not because of the tooth itself but because of other reasons, such as gum disease or, scientifically speaking, gingivitis. So when we lose our tooth, usually our tooth looks every which way normal, sometimes in perfect shape. When the tooth is pulled out, the shape is intact, and the color is pearly white—meaning, in perfect condition. But it says goodbye to the owner with tears in its eyes. Actually, the tears are in the owner's eyes. Now we lose our tooth due to the problem of the surrounding structures, not the tooth itself.

Dentists were busy in the past because of decayed teeth. Now they are busier than before because of gum disease. In the past, when a dentist extracted a tooth, especially if it was a molar tooth, the dentist was going to be in trouble because it was so hard. Literally, they had to sweat it out profusely. Now it is so easy to pull out because it is almost already out. Just pull it out. That's all. In the old days, when one or two teeth were decayed and pulled out, then the dentist would grind the neighboring teeth with no mercy at all and put something called "bridge" on the top of it. Now instead of the bridge, dentists put or screw in something called "implant." So the adjacent teeth are saved from the no-mercy grinding. But whether it is a crown or implant, a person who has no experience has no idea what other people are going through.

So next, I'm going to discuss why the perfect-looking teeth are saying goodbye to the owner in tears. I already gave the explanation that it is due to the failure of the surrounding supporting tissues, including the bones. This time, I'm going to explain the reason for the failure of the surrounding tissue and, at the same time, the prevention of the problem.

Our teeth and gums are well protected by our own lips from bad temperatures, especially cold; dryness; excessive external force; etc. Most of the time, our teeth are hiding behind the lips. Once they show up, they disappear immediately, like a shy young girl, except only when we talk, yawn, or sing, etc.

Why is it such a hard task to keep our teeth and gums clean even though we brush our teeth three times a day or more and gargle with a very expensive antiseptic solution as many as possible? A few months ago, I read in the newspaper and in the medical journal that brushing the teeth can only clean the inside of our mouth at 25 percent, and the rest remains the same before and after. I absolute agree with this. This is the reason why.

These are the three most important causes of gum disease and halitosis.

First, **we have the most ideal environment in our mouth for the germs, bacteria, viruses, fungi, etc., to grow and prosper.** Like anywhere else in our body, our mouth is the best, if not one of the best, place that germs want to stay and grow. The mouth has the most ideal temperature and moisture for germs to grow. On top of these two favorable conditions, the oxygen supply is blocked most of the time, but there is an unlimited supply of oxygen when we open up our mouth—which makes it an ideal place both for aerobic (needing oxygen to survive) and anaerobic (not requiring oxygen to survive) organisms to grow. No matter how cold or hot outside, the inside of our mouth remains a perfect, calm, and peaceful environment. **In reality, our mouth is filled with all kinds of germs already. So if there is any kind of injuries in our mouth, the germs will grow like wildfire.** This wildfire will continue day and night, whether we are asleep or awake, until it destroys completely the surrounding structures of our teeth.

Second, we are injuring our mouth, specifically our gums, all the time. If you think eating food itself does not cause any injury to our gums, that's a big misunderstanding. If you look under the microscope, numerous injuries occur while eating. That's all the germs need because germs are so tiny to invade into our skin, the barrier. There are so many ways we injure our mouth. There is one way to injure our mouth without thinking. People living in cold climate have tendencies to eat or drink hot food. That kind of eating habit can give first-degree, or sometimes second-degree, burn inside our mouth. We do not have a good distribution of sensory nerve cells in our mouth, particularly in the gums, that we do not feel that much of pain as we are supposed to. There is another way. This is iatrogenic and self-induced. It is toothpick. And a detailed explanation comes soon.

Third and the most important, the frame or the architecture of our teeth itself is the problem. Our teeth or its structure itself can be one of the root causes of gum disease. It is inevitable to have a gum disease. If we look at our teeth very closely, the more you look at close to the root, the tooth becomes slender. Anatomically, the tooth looks like an athlete with wide shoulders and a slender waist. It does not look like a fat guy with a belly wider than his shoulders. A little bit of different-but-similar-looking teeth of fourteen, sometimes sixteen on the top and the bottom, altogether twenty-eight or thirty-two teeth, arranged side by side and next to each other, are sitting inside our mouth. So quite naturally, there is no space between the shoulder area, but there are plenty of spaces in the waist area. I call this space "the triangle of death."

Below this triangle of death, below the gums, the root of the tooth is planted into the bones of the maxilla on the top and the mandible at the bottom. In this triangle of death, when we eat any food, the particle of the food sticks in with ease, most of the times tiny and small in size but occasionally big one. And whatever the reason is, when and if an infection sets in, a few of the abundant germs follow in, and our gum disease starts. Then when the infection goes down and down and finally the bone gets infected, the normal-looking and perfect shape of our tooth has to leave home sweet home. There is no choice. Most of the time, the triangle of death collects the well-grinded minute food particles, but sometimes a big piece of meat gets stuck in and tries to take a small step to achieve the giant goal to destroy our valuable assets.

However, with good brushes and excellent toothpaste, we can clean the front and the back sides of our teeth. And we can perhaps kill all the germs inside our mouth with a powerful and expensive antiseptic liquid. There is no way we can reach in and clean this triangle of death as much as we want. No matter how hard we might try, it is impossible to clean this area of death, and it will be not much different before and after all the cleaning efforts we put in. And remember that we are cleaning this area at 25 percent only, except with the method that I'm about to recommend, which will achieve almost 100 percent of our goal to clean the triangle of death.

In other words, no matter how desperately we brush our teeth and so on, we go to bed with almost the same condition, having not able to clean the area where cleaning is most desperately needed. You may feel fresh after brushing your teeth. That's all you achieved, feeling fresh. The dirty area you wanted to clean still remains dirty or not changed.

We need to change this! We need to add the thing I'm recommending. In fact, even while we are cleaning, the gum disease in the triangle of death, which is the worst area we have to focus on, still continues to be the same at most or gets worse. Cleaning this triangle of death is the best way to eliminate gum disease, also known as gingivitis, and halitosis as well. And the best way to achieve this goal will soon come out.

Before we get to the conclusion, I'd like to talk about a very small but also very important thing. As we all know that not only all the teeth look not the same but also their functions. Each tooth looks different and functions different.

What I'm going to discuss here is about our canine teeth, especially the ones on the top on both sides, right and left. Canine teeth? Do we need them? Yeah, we need them for cosmetic reason. In the animal kingdom, for the predators—like tigers, lions, wolves, bears, etc.—these are vital to hunt other animals. They use their canine teeth to kill other animals. Of course, Count Dracula needed strong canines for his survival. We all know the reason why we all want to keep distance from him. Then why do we need the canines? We do not need them for survival, unless we are descendants of Count Dracula. For cosmetic reason, we need our canine teeth. All cosmetic reasons. You will notice them immediately if you see a person who lost these two. There is a distinct difference in the appearance of the person between before and after. As a matter of fact, we do not realize them while we have them, but we recognize them immediately after we lose them. Furthermore, people and your friends may not recognize you in the crowd when you lost your canines.

Have you ever seen a pulled canine? If not, any photos? Among our teeth, it is the longest one. This root of canines stretches to or passes the edge of our nares. It is so important when it is in place because it maintains and supports the better half of our face from being sunken. We look young and handsome or beautiful. I hope there is no one who believes that even after we pulled out such a big structure, we would look as good as when we had it in place. When the canines are gone, the area where the root of the canines were located will go down just a little bit that we all are going to look like the face of the Wicked Witch of the West, regardless if we are a man or a woman. To our most sensitive organ in our body, our eyes, "just a little bit" makes a huge difference. A person who is aged with wrinkles all over the face may look old but may maintain the way they look when they were young; thus, people will recognize them easily. But a person who lost both canines, no matter how many times they got Botox injections, may look young without wrinkles on the face, but even their best friends would not recognize them, even if they pass by in a close distance. So no matter how old you may be, by keeping the face of your young age with help of your canines, when you happened to meet your old friend on the street, you can smile wide from ear to ear and become a competent old man without covering your mouth with your hand. If you do not want to cover the bottom half of your face, you have to keep your canines until the day you die. No matter how old you may be, if you want to show your handsome face of your young age to your grandson, granddaughter, great-grandson, great-granddaughter and so on, you have to keep your canines to the best of your ability. Especially for all the ladies, keep the fact in mind all the time that keeping those two canines will be far superior to multiple Botox injections, face-lifts, etc. This is not a threatening statement to justify the function of canines. Just ask your dentist. The answer is not very far.

One question, how about an implant? The answer is right there if you look at an implant when it is ready to go inside your mouth. Google it and look at the entire shape of the implant, especially on the part of the root. It is not as long or as thick as a real tooth. It does not replace the natural shape of our real canines.

Let's go back to the cleaning of the triangle of death. What if we clean the area with toothpicks? Apparently, using a toothpick is the worst solution for this problem. A toothpick is one of the worst, if not the worst, enemies of our gums. The sharp front of the toothpick will poke, scratch, and cut our defenseless, innocent gums at will and introduce a safe house to the ever-so-happy multiple germs because the toothpicks cannot see. They are blind. They do not know what is ahead, and they do not know what they are doing, which means they will do a very nasty damage to our gums without any guilty feeling because they do not have a brain or heart. If you want to or have to use a toothpick, then use it gently with extreme caution only on the front and back sides of the teeth and never poke it into the triangle of death. That's when you injure your helpless and priceless gums.

Another question, how about dental floss? It is not as dangerous as toothpicks, but it is dangerous. Recent study shows there is not much difference between them. It is the same that they cannot see what they are doing. A floss can cut tofu or hot dog with ease as a toothpick can cut through tofu or hot dog. Do you think your infected, diseased gums are stronger than tofu or hot dog? I hope not. If you floss the infected gum in the triangle of death, the result would be the same or similar at best as toothpick. When you do it, the same as with toothpick, do it gently with extreme caution.

There is one thing you have to keep in mind. When you use the floss, you have to make sure you are alone. Make sure no one is around you. Not even in front of your family or very close friends. It will be a big mistake if you floss in front of them because they are your spouse, parents, siblings, relatives, or close friends. Apparently, they are the people who want to see your handsome or beautiful face instead of your less-than-handsome or less-than-beautiful face. The reason is when you floss, your face turns from handsome to less than handsome or from beautiful to less than beautiful in a split second of time.

Not too long ago, in the *Family Feud*, one of my favorite game shows, there was an interesting question: "What is something that a man should not do in front of his wife or girlfriend?" There were seven answers on the board, but I only remember five of them. I do not remember which one is number 1 or which one is number 7. This is what I remember: do not fart, do not burp at the dinner table, do not curse, do not put your pants down in front of her or do not show your most valuable part, and do not floss in front of her after dinner. I was so glad that there are some people in this world who have the same opinion or feeling as I have.

Now here's the conclusion or the answer to how to clean up the triangle of death in our mouth. It took a long time to come to this point, trying not to offend the feelings of good people. Here's how to clean up the triangle of death. First, it has to be safe so that it does not cause any damage to the gums to prevent easy access for the nasty germs to cross the barrier. Second, it has to be effective. It has to be proven effective. I'm going to show how to fulfill these two conditions simultaneously. Third, the price has to be reasonable. With one condition: you have to continue what you are doing and what you have been doing. Continue what you do. Do not stop.

I want you to add what I'm suggesting to what you are doing. I'm going to introduce to you a small equipment that some of you already know and are using already. It is known to you as WaterPik or water floss. But the name of the product is water floss, and the name of the company is WaterPik.

Of course, you can find it at any pharmacies and Costco as well. If something or anything is available at Costco, I recommend Costco. I explained the reason already, and you know that I did not receive anything from Costco. A few months ago, I bought a new one for myself because I needed a new one. The regular price was seventy-nine dollars, but with manufacturer's rebate, I only paid fifty-nine dollars.

Not many people are using it. If I talk to people, about two out of ten are currently using it. It rarely goes over three. I do not know who invented it or what company did the research and develop. But I think it's worth to give a Nobel Prize. Probably because it looks and works like the "water gun" in the dentist's chair, the Nobel Committee decided not to award it. Actually, it copied the main function of the water gun at a dental office.

The user's manual is in the box, but it is very simple and easy to use it. The main mechanism of the function of this equipment is cleaning with forceful water. It cleans with forceful water, like a dentist does with their water gun. We can control and adjust the force and velocity of the water. If you run it with too much force, you can damage the gums. This is the only one that requires caution. I always adjust the speed of the water in the middle. Naturally, the water temperature needs to be not too hot or cold. Just warm is enough, like our body temperature. If you keep your mouth closed while you are using it, the water will remain inside your mouth. You can do it before you go to bed. Sometimes, some of the very smart people would mix a little bit of salt or antiseptic liquid products to the water, such as Listerine.

Before long, you will get your true smell. It will come back to you. Pretty soon, the gum disease no longer will bother you. And the decomposing food particles will disappear from your triangle of death. Then the bad smell that bothers you and others that bother you will say goodbye to you as long as you use this equipment. And the smell of your own body, the true smell, comes back. When you wake up in the morning with your own smell, you will realize that I told you the truth, the best truth.

Again, I did not receive anything from this magnificent company of WaterPik. Simply, I do not know them, and they do not know me.

CHAPTER 16

Five Hundred

It happened about one year before the presidential election. It was November of 1999. There was a small boat accident in the sea between Miami and Cuba, which nobody paid attention to. A few people drowned, but most of them were rescued. It was nothing new and nothing surprising. It happens all the time. It was close to the beach of Miami. It was dark, but people in the boat were able to see the light on the building or in the street when it sank. But because of this small accident at the sea, almost at the beach of Miami, the history of America had changed, which means the history of the entire world had changed as well.

The boat was too old and small to carry all the people on board and started sinking. In the boat, there was a young woman with a seven-year-old son who wanted to join her family in Miami and who was one of the drowned. Because she gave her son the only life jacket given to her by the crew of the boat. And she herself swam, but she did not make it to the beach. She wanted to come to America, the land of opportunities, like many others.

In this world, we all know that even if it is exactly the same action or behavior, the outcome or consequence would be entirely different or sometimes exactly opposite. For example, if we kill a person in the street, we become a murderer. But if we kill a person or as many as we can in a battlefield, we become a hero in our town, and our president will give us the special Medal of Honor with a big ceremony at the White House.

Though it is not the same, a similar interpretation or result can occur in immigration issues. Crossing the border either by sea or by land, which are exact same actions, will be treated in an entirely opposite way. If you cross the border without a legal paper from Mexico, you will be treated like a criminal, as an illegal alien. You will be locked up like a criminal and deported eventually. But if you cross the border—in this case and most of the time by sea—from Cuba, even though you have no legal paper whatsoever, you will be granted political asylum. And you will be given an American citizenship eventually. These are exactly the same actions with exactly opposite outcomes.

Not too long ago, when there was an uprising against the Communist Chinese government in Tiananmen Square, there was also an uprising among the Chinese in the many cities of America. Many of them—students, tourists, businesspersons, etc.—went to the White House to demonstrate. During this short time of uprising, the Chinese were given the same right or privilege as Cubans have. They could apply for political asylum.

So in the case of Cubans, they have to cross the sea, which is not a big deal in terms of the distance and time. But if they get caught in the sea, they are illegal and will be locked up and deported. If they step even one foot on the beach, even though it is just one step on the American soil of sand beach, they will be granted political asylum and guaranteed to become American citizens soon.

It is real close between Cuba and Miami. In a good sunny day, you can see Cuba from Key West of Florida. It could be close and very far at the same time. It is close because you can see Cuba with your own naked eyes and it takes less than an hour in a speedy boat.

It could be very far because you have to risk your, life like this young boy's mom. On November of 1999, this young woman, raising a seven-year-old boy after being divorced, decided to move to America and join her family in Miami, Florida. She escaped Cuba with people who were in similar situation and with the same goal. But because there were too many people on a small boat or the boat was too old, the boat started sinking after they successfully avoided a Cuban naval ship and almost avoided the US Coast Guard.

Miraculously, the boy was able to land on the beach, but the young mom did not make it to the beach. The young boy who lost his mom began his American dream under the care of his uncle, growing up with his cousins. But his American dream came to a screeching halt when his father showed up out of nowhere and claimed to have his son back with him in Cuba.

In the beginning, it took the shape of a family feud that a father is looking for his long-lost child. Then it became an international legal dispute. Who had the legal custody? The father wanted to have his son back to his custody, and the boy's uncle refused to send him back, stating it was the boy's mother's wish or dream for him to remain in America and keep the dream alive. So it became a court case from Miami to Atlanta, where the higher court is. And finally, even Fidel Castro became involved, who threatened to bring the case to an international court and humiliate America internationally. The court also leaned toward the father, who had the ultimate custody of the boy, his son.

The relatives of the boy, uncles and aunts, became desperate as well. Numerous Cubans in Miami were also on the side of the boy's uncles and aunts and went out on the street and in front of the court every day and began to demonstrate.

Despite the international turmoil, the presidential election continued to come close. In the primary elections of each parties, the Democrats elected the current vice president, Al Gore, as their candidate while the Republicans elected a lot-less-known Texas governor, George W. Bush, son of former president George H. W. Bush.

In the year of a presidential election, potential candidates would announce their intentions as early as possible, but most of them would announce their candidacies in the early part of the year because the campaign for the primary election would begin very early. By the time the primary election is over and by the end of June and each party would have nominated their candidates in their conventions, we would know who is going to be the next president of United States of America, one of the parties' nominees.

In the year 2000 presidential election, unless there was a major upset or unexpected event, it was Al Gore who would become the next president of the United States. Al Gore was Al Gore, the current vice president and the vice president of one of the most successful presidents in recent memory, Bill Clinton, except for one scandal, in my opinion. The only disadvantage of Al Gore was the fact that the previous two terms of the president for eight years was by the Democrats, who was Bill Clinton.

On the other hand, George W. Bush, son of the former president George H. W. Bush, was the nominee. Actually, his younger brother, Jeb Bush, the current governor of Florida, was more famous and more presidential than him. But George became famous or got notoriety due to what he did as Texas governor, although he was still the sitting governor of Texas. He did not allow or give any commutation to a death row inmate despite the plea from a well-known religious group or people, even the pope in the Vatican. Like a leader in the past, he became famous by killing people, and killing even more people after he became the leader of the free world.

By the way, the election of the president of the USA is done by indirect voting system. It has been like that since the birth of America. The rests are direct voting system, such as of the senators, congressmen and women, governors, mayors, etc.

For the president, the citizens elect the electoral college of each state in November, who then elects the president in January. But it is interesting and strange to see that the candidate who gets one more vote will get the entire electoral college votes of any particular state. Sometimes, it is strange to see a candidate who receives less votes than the other candidate wins and becomes the elected president of the US. The number of electoral college of each state is determined by the number of citizens, i.e., voters, living in the state, i.e., the number of congressmen of the state. So the total number of the electoral college is the total number of congressman of each state plus two times fifty (or the number of senators of each state times fifty).

The state of California, which is the most heavily populated state, has fifty-five electoral college votes. And the state of Texas has thirty-eight. Then New York and Florida each has twenty-nine votes.

The exact number of electoral college votes varies just a little bit on each election, depending on the population changes. According to the record, on the last election, the number of total electoral college votes was 538. Any candidate who goes over half of the above number wins the election and becomes the next president of United States. Sometimes and not infrequently, a candidate who loses in total votes can win in electoral college votes. In some states, they win the electoral college votes in a narrow margin, and in some other states, they lose in a wide margin. Then the person wins the election but loses the presidency. The loser becomes the winner, and the winner becomes the loser. That's the irony of the presidential election of the USA.

But it does not matter, whether direct or indirect, who is the winner or the loser. Any election in any country will be determined by the amount of money. If someone says he can run a campaign and win an election without spending any money, the person must be from the other planet, not from earth. In any country, whoever has more money or whichever party has more money will win the election. Particularly in the American election, you have to have money.

However, let's put aside the money factor. Then what is the next most important deciding factor in the American election? Generally speaking, the candidate from the Republican Party has to win any election whatsoever because of the abovementioned factor. No question about that. But the candidate from the Democratic Party has a good chance or better chance to win any election also. What is the reason? How is it possible? This is the second most, maybe the most, important deciding factor in American election. At least up until now and quite some time in the near future, it will continue the trend quite a while.

Yes, the deciding votes in American election is and has to be Black votes, in my opinion. Are you out of your mind? Will only 10 percent of the entire population decide the result of the election? Yes, when the Black voters come out and vote, the Democratic candidate wins. And if not, the Republican candidate wins. Plain and simple. If the Democratic candidate knows or masters how to mobilize Black votes, they win. If not, the answer is plain and simple. The Republican Party wins.

That's why the Republicans are trying desperately to make it extremely difficult for the Black people to come out and vote. If you have any question or doubt about this reality, just go back to the previous presidential election up to President Reagan. This is the truth and the reality of American politics until now and quite some time in the future. In the general election, not to mention about the in-between elections which show far less participation than in the general election, only more or less than half of us go out to vote, and a little bit more than half will decide who will be the next president of the US and the leader of the free world. That is the reason why the 10 percent Black population is so important. It is almost automatic that if they stay home, the Republicans win. If they come out and vote, the Democrats win.

If this formula stays the same, it will remain the same pattern until we see a different pattern for a long time coming. First, let's look at the immediate past.

Let's start with President Obama. He had no problem mobilizing the Black voters. On top of that, he did not do anything negative against the Whites and other minorities. But on his second term, he almost lost the election at the first debate. His opponent's popularity went up so high after the first debate that he needed the help of Joe Biden, who saved him with the one and only vice presidential debate. Even now, many Republicans are claiming they lost the game that they almost won, which I agree. They were celebrating already even though there were two more debates remaining and there was a long time left until election day. As a matter of fact, I think Mr. Mitt Romney was and still is the best Republican candidate who lost to a Democratic candidate in recent memory. It is particularly true if you look at what's going on in the White House since 2018. In danger of losing to Mr. Romney, who do you think saved Mr. Obama? Guess who? Black voters and Mr. Joe Biden.

Next, let's talk about President Bush, the son. Black voters did not come out and vote for the Democratic candidate. I do not even remember the name of the Democratic candidate, even though I voted for him.

Next is President Bill Clinton. He is the genius of the geniuses in politics, who mastered the truth of the 10 percent. When he went to a Black community or church and met the people, he did not shake hands. He hugged everyone. It did not matter to him whether they were men or women or young or old; he hugged everyone. That's why he defeated the current incumbent president of the US. He is the one and only genius in politics. He turned around the economy and successfully avoided the Republicans' desperate attempt to impeach him. Only if he did not have the Lewinski affair, he would be one of the top 3 or top 5 most famous past presidents in the US history.

And there is President Jimmy Carter, who is Mr. Nice Guy, a Sunday school teacher, and a Bible study teacher from the South, State of Georgia. Unfortunately, he became a one-term president because of Ronald Reagan. I'm going to talk about Mr. Reagan more on the chapter "Heimlich Maneuver."

So we elect our president, the leader of the free world, with more or less than half of all the voters. And when we have a strong independent candidate, then a little bit more or sometimes less than half of the voters will elect the president of the USA. Half of the half, i.e., one fourth, of the voters will elect or decide who is going to be the next president. This is the reality, the true face, and the current address of the American election, which has to be changed one way or another.

It does not sound right to me that the leader of the country is determined by the support of a little bit more or sometimes less than 25 percent of all the voters. Wake up, America! We can do better than this. We have to do better than this. A percentage of 25 of us elect our president, the leader of our country and the leader of the free world. This does not make any sense to me. Does it make sense to you? Oh no, not to me.

Let's go back to the young boy. In the court battle, the argument was leaning toward the father, who legally had the ultimate custody of the son. So the Cubans in Miami and entire Florida and the entire country who supported for the boy to remain in the US and continue the American dream went out to the street and also started talking and pleading to the politicians—senators, congress-men, governor—and the White House. As the presidential election came closer, they sat down and talked and pleaded to Al Gore. But Al Gore himself, even though he was the vice president of the US and had a very high chance to be the next president, could not break the law of the land. And furthermore, he himself had to follow and reinforce the law.

Finally, the Federal Court of Atlanta, Georgia, decided in favor of the boy's father and ordered to hand over the boy to his father. The Cubans and the family refused to accept the verdict, and the tension grew between the two groups—the law enforcement agency, i.e., the government, and the Cubans. The law enforcement agency of the government, i.e., FBI, gave the ultimatum to the Cubans and the family and set the date to hand over the boy to them. The family and the Cubans knew that the FBI would take the boy by force when and if they would not hand him over. And so they organized a group of people, like bodyguards, to protect the boy twenty-four hours.

But on a hot summer night, heavily armed FBI agents sur-rounded and raided the house and took the sleeping boy by force and gave him to the waiting father within a few hours. Everything was done as quick as lightning. In the middle of the night, when everybody was tired and asleep, a group of heavily armed FBI agents rushed into the house where the boy was sleeping, took the boy away from the bodyguards at gunpoint, and delivered the boy to his father even before the sunrise.

All the Cubans knew the next morning that the boy was long gone. They, the angry Cubans, started swearing at the government and ultimately at Al Gore that they would not show up in November of that year or that they would vote for Al Gore's opponent. Yes, you guessed right, at the presidential election.

If this incident did not happen or happened after November, we would have Al Gore, not Bush, as the next president of the USA in that election. The reason is that most of the Cubans would usually vote for a Democratic candidate in the presidential election. They turned their back against Al Gore, either by staying at home on election day or voting for his opponent, Mr. Bush, in retaliation.

But not many people, including myself and especially Al Gore's camp, considered or realized that this small event, i.e., incident, would affect the outcome of the general election because major opinion polls showed that Mr. Gore was way ahead of Mr. Bush. So the day of destiny arrived.

The presidential election in America always occurs on the first Tuesday of November. We are going through this interesting phenomenon every day, which is the sun rises in the east and sets in the west. But on this particular November day, we are not just going through it. We feel it to the deepest part of our skin, which is the sun rises from the east and goes down to the west.

We have three different time zones in America, excluding Alaska and Hawaii. When people in New York or Detroit wake up at seven o'clock in the morning, the people in Seattle and Los Angeles are still fast asleep at four o'clock in the morning. At nine thirty every morning, when the New York stock market opens up, the Dow Jones Industrial Average collapses, and the retirement funds plummet to the bottom, as in one Black Friday. The people in Los Angeles do not know anything about their retirement funds because they were still in bed, sleeping like a baby. When the Detroit Tigers play in Los Angeles, the game starts at seven or seven thirty in the evening in local time, but it is ten or ten thirty in the evening in Detroit. So quite naturally, a person like me has to stay up after midnight, and if the game goes into extra inning, I'm in trouble the following day, especially if the Tigers lose. I'll be suffering from major league sleep deprivation syndrome the next day because I do not like my team to lose in the first place. I only had a few hours of sleep.

Let's go back to the election day. People in the East Coast vote first, specifically three hours earlier. And the voting ends three hours earlier than the people in the West Coast. In reality, while the people in the West Coast are still voting, the voting in the East Coast is already done and closed. And due to the advancement in the computer system, the results are coming out on major news channels while people in the West Coast are still voting. Sometimes or theoretically, we know the result even while people are still voting. Why? Because other than time zone, there is another factor.

Usually but not all the time, those states in the coastal area, East Coast and West Coast, are voting for the Democratic candidate—especially New York, New Jersey, Massachusetts, West Virginia, Florida, California, Washington, Oregon, etc.—and those states in between go to the Republican candidate. So by the time we know about the results of New York, New Jersey, Massachusetts, South and North Carolina, Florida, and some swing states like Michigan and Ohio, we can safely say who would be the next president of the USA, even though the people in the West Coast are still voting. Many times, the major news media would announce the winner before the official result comes out, the so-called presumptive winner, by the time we know the results of Michigan and Ohio. I can go to bed around ten o'clock or eleven o'clock in the evening knowing the presumptive winner, who would be the confirmed winner. Almost all the time, the name of the presumptive and official winner does not change. I had to say "almost" because something happened the other way on that election.

Actually, on that election night, NBC, one of the three major news media, announced around ten o'clock in the evening that Al Gore was the winner. Usually, about ten o'clock in the evening of the election, we would know the result when the presumptive winner is announced, and it would become official the next morning. Of course, it is not official. It is presumptive. But you know what would happen the next morning. Certainly, I took it the way they said and the way I heard. I was not the only one or one of the few who took it the way it was. I went to bed around ten o'clock in the evening after I heard the presumptive winner's name, assuming that he, Al Gore, would be my president for the next four years, hopefully next eight years. But the next morning, when I woke up and turned on the TV, the news anchors were talking somewhat different. They said there was no official winner in the election. There was no official winner because no one crossed the magic number of 270 of electoral college. Because there was no winner in Florida. They were still counting the votes. Actually, they were recounting. And the number that was coming out said that George Bush was ahead by the thinnest margin.

The Republicans were already celebrating. Celebrating? Without an official announcement? By the time the recount was about to be over, Mr. Bush was ahead by approximately five hundred votes in Florida. The Democrats were demanding to take the case to the Supreme Court, but the Republicans were smiling big.

First, at the state level, who was the sitting governor of Florida? The answer was Jeb Bush, who had the same last name with George and is the younger brother of George.

The most important question: "Who is the secretary of state of Florida?" This time, her last name was not important. That person was a lady, and we did not need to know her last name. What was the most important at this juncture was what she was, not who she was. This is what she was. She was the one, as secretary of state, who oversaw and supervised the election process. And as long as her candidate was ahead, she would never change the number of votes. She would never look at anywhere else. She would never make any decision going against her party's candidate.

Then the result went to the Supreme Court. At the Supreme Court, the decision would be handed out by the nine Supreme Court judges, of whom four were on the Republican side and four were on the Democratic side. Then who was the one? Who was the deciding vote? He was the chief justice at that time, Antonin Scalia, who was nominated by Ronald Reagan and confirmed by the senate. If the result came from the Lower Court with Mr. Bush ahead, he would never vote against the party that made him to be the chief justice. So it took more than a month for the Supreme Court to hand down the decision that Mr. Bush was the winner of Florida's electoral college vote and, as a result, announced that Mr. Bush was the next president of the USA.

Just before the Supreme Court came down with the decision, for which Mr. Bush was so happy to wait, Mr. Gore made his own personal decision and made the announcement—which is definitely one of the best speeches made by any politician ever made for the sake of national unity—in front of his supporters and fellow Democrats who urged him to fight until the end, regardless of the Supreme Court decision. He said, "It's time for me to go." He was thinking of his fellow Americans, not himself. Thus, for eight years, we had a president who was thinking only of himself and a few others rather than his fellow Americans, the citizens of the United States of America.

As it turned out, this was the moment that the American history forever changed because we all know what happened to our retirement fund and entire economy. And the history of the world forever changed because we all know what happened in 9/11, followed by the Iraq War. How many innocent people died, both Americans and Iraqis? Not only the American economy but also the world economy went down the drain together. Many peoples' businesses and houses never returned. A few of my acquaintances went bankrupt and disappeared from the community. Yes, five hundred votes had changed the history of America and ultimately the history of the world. And you know the rest of the story. How many young Americans died and were injured? The numbers are staggering, when we include the number of Iraqi people who died and were injured. You know what happened in Iraq, and you know what happened to your retirement fund, i.e., your personal economy, and the national economy and the world economy.

That is the reason why we have to vote. It does not matter whether you are Left or Right, Progressive or Conservative, Democrat or Republican, Socialist or Capitalist, Black or White or Brown, young or old, ladies or gentlemen. You have to vote. You have to express who you are and what your opinion is. The best way to do it as a citizen of America is to *vote*! You have to vote for you. And you have to vote for your family, for your country—the United States of America—and for the world, for god's sake!

By the way, the young boy's name is Elián González. He is not a boy anymore. He is a man now, who is older than twenty.

CHAPTER 17

Heimlich Maneuver

When we eat, sometimes the food we just ate gets lost in the right direction and ends up at the wrong area. We call this event "choking." As a result, the food, small or big, sometimes can block the air circulation to our entire body, especially to the brain. If such a dangerous condition lasts longer than four to six minutes, it will leave a permanent brain damage and ultimately result in death if the oxygen supply remains shut down. In such an imminent danger of life or death, there is a maneuver available that makes it to turn our lives from death to a new life.

What is it? What is it that is giving us a new life? It is written above, Heimlich maneuver.

Henry Heimlich, M. D., the creator of this maneuver, was born in the city of Wilmington, Delaware, on February 3, 1920. He is living in Cincinnati, Ohio, and still very healthy. In 1974, he introduced this maneuver for the first time through the American Heart Association. Ever since, this maneuver has been spread out to the entire world, and we do not know how many peoples' lives have been saved because we do not have the official data for this particular area. We do not know how many people have been given a new life. He should have been awarded a Nobel Prize a long time ago, but there is no official report yet.

Anyway, before the Heimlich maneuver was introduced, when a piece of food blocks the airway, people used to blow hard on the back of the victim with the palm of the hand over and over. We call this the back blow method. Currently, the American Red Cross recommends and teaches first responders and medical professionals to attempt the back blow method twice or thrice and then to attempt the Heimlich maneuver if the back blow method is unsuccessful. So the dispute and conflict between the American Red Cross and Dr. Heimlich still continues because the American Red Cross insists to attempt the back blow method first, followed by Heimlich maneuver, and Dr. Heimlich continues to preach to attempt the Heimlich maneuver first. According to Dr. Heimlich, if we blow hard the back of a choking victim, due to the pain and loud noise, it is human nature, i.e., physiological response or the reflex of our body, to inhale, which will create a negative pressure in our chest cavity, which will make the foreign body go down farther.

And the dispute continues, but neither side is going to prevail. The reason is we cannot perform a research about which method is superior to the other. Maybe we can do animal study. But we cannot experiment this to a human being. There will be no human volunteers for this research. No, absolutely not. Who will volunteer for this? At what price? You? Or me? No, not you or not me. So the dispute continues. No one knows when it will end.

But you will find out which side I am standing with if and when you finish reading this chapter. You will get the answer if you continue to read. It is up to you which method you apply and which side you stand with. What is important is you have to save a choking person. It does not matter which method you apply. You have no time to think which one you are going to choose, not even one second for this, because one second might make the difference between life or the other. You know what I mean.

The core content of the Heimlich maneuver is abdominal thrust. Unfortunately, we call a person a choking victim if the person is on the crossroad of life or death due to a foreign body, usually food, that is stuck in their airway. Instantaneously and aggressively, you put a strong pressure on the middle portion between the belly button and the lower portion of the sternum. The most common position is like a bear hugging a tree. You position yourself at the back of a choking victim. And then you put a sudden pressure toward yourself as if you're having a convulsion. If the choking victim happens to be too big for you to grab from behind, you can put the person on the hard floor and go on the top of the person with both hands together and then do the same. In case of children, you sit down on a chair, put the victim on your lap, and do the same. When you hold your hand together, put your stronger hand—righties use right hand and lefties use left hand—ninety degrees toward the victim. The thumb and index side should be toward the victim, which will deliver the maximum blow, not the palm side which is flat and which will not give the maximum blow.

In a peaceful moment, when you go to a good restaurant with your family or friends having a quality time, a person next to your table might suddenly become a choking victim. When a piece of meat enters into the wrong way and blocks the airway, usually the person does his best to remove it to the best of their ability and then, if unsuccessful, will make a strange noise and then grab their neck with both hands and try to stand up but will be unable to do it. That is when the person next to the victim recognizes what happened. The person will witness the typical posture of a choking victim, with both hands grabbing their neck and face turning blue or dark blue, even black. This is the moment of truth. At this crucial moment, somebody or anybody nearby should calmly go around the victim's back and perform the Heimlich maneuver. You will be successful to save the person's life. I guarantee you the color of the victim's face would come back to normal, and the person would talk again, saying, "Thank you, thank you, thank you." They would begin their second life thanking you for everything every day for the rest of their life. This is not what I said. Dr. Heimlich said that.

But at this crucial moment, if everybody becomes panicky and confused, you know the rest of the story. Even if an ambulance and the first responders show up, after four to six minutes, the story ends. However, if you count calmly, "One and two and three…" and so on, you could do what you have to do one at a time. Four to six minutes is not so short and is not going to be that short as you might think. It is long enough to save a person's life. But if you are in a panic and not doing what you are supposed to do, like anything else, the time flies. It is as simple as that. Again, calmly step to the back of the victim and perform the Heimlich maneuver. Be calm outside, even though you are panicky inside.

Even though in the book, they advise to do it up to five times and think about the next step or something else, you have to do it more than five times if necessary. The American Red Cross advises five times of the back blow method, followed by five times of the Heimlich maneuver. And then we have to decide whether we have to go to the next step if Heimlich maneuver does not solve the problem.

In case we fail to bring up the blocking foreign body, the story does not end at that point. The moment we move to the next step after five or more attempts of the Heimlich maneuver, the purpose changes from the removal of the foreign body to saving a human life, which is the ultimate goal of everything we do. Keep the person alive until the first responder shows up and takes over and continues what you were doing. We have to move to CPR (cardiopulmonary resuscitation). As soon as you have made the decision to move to CPR, you tell a person next to you to call an ambulance. And then you start the CPR, by one man or two men, until the first responder arrives.

So far, this was an example of a choking victim and about what you can do. But if you happened to see an unconscious person in the dark corner of a street, you have to shake the person first to see if the person is sleeping or unconscious. If unconscious, tell the bystanders to call an ambulance or call 911 and start CPR immediately.

But one thing is clear. No matter what the outcome might have been, even if the result is negative or bad, the performer is not responsible for the bad outcome. Successful or not, the performer is not responsible. The performer is protected by the law, which is the Good Samaritan law. Do not worry about bad outcome. It is not your fault. It is the victim's fault for the bad luck.

Let's go back to the story of mine. I jumped into a society with which I had little knowledge and absolutely no experience at all. It is like jumping into the Pacific Ocean for a person who never learned swimming. All I had was the fact that I was young and had blind courage. I was afraid of nothing. I had no doubt in my mind that I would succeed in my life. But I did not have the slightest idea that life is not easy and this much difficult.

At the time I came to America, Ronald Reagan was the president. He was somebody who failed as an actor and as a husband. But he was very successful as a politician. He was someone who beat up the sitting president and then became the newly elected president.

The country appeared calm outside, but internally, turmoil was brewing real hard. Unexpectedly and suddenly, the political environment changed from Jimmy Carter to Ronald Reagan, from a Democratic president to a Republican president, and from Socialism to Capitalism. America needed sufficient time to change. It was too short for the entire country to change from one philosophy to another. Four years was too short. It was like the Pacific Ocean, peaceful superficially but turbulence was brewing at the bottom.

The enormous change that Mr. Reagan was about to bring to the entire country was about to start. Particularly after the First World War and the Second World War, the entire country was suffering from high unemployment and deepened poverty, for there were a lot of soldiers who were released from the military forces looking for jobs. To solve these serious and significant national issues, naturally the Democratic Party's Socialistic approach attracted majority of the people as a more viable solution. Now the government became the center of the solution and the problem simultaneously. The government became the leader fighting the ever-growing poverty and the biggest employee. One after another, the government made a big announcement of enormous projects which would employ the young, poor, and unemployed, who were pouring out into the society from the military.

Mr. Reagan became a rising star in the Republican Party, pointing out government bureaucracy. And wherever he went, he laid out his agenda and solution. He emphasized a "small but efficient government and yet with a strong military."

A lot of Democrats crossed over the party line and gave their votes to Mr. Reagan. Actually, Mr. Reagan started his political career as a Democrat. So he knew the Democratic Party's absurdity better than most of us and took advantage of it. Those Democrats who betrayed the Democratic Party got a new name, Reagan Democrats. Many of the Democrats who made their fortune through Democratic Socialistic governmental project gave their soul to Mr. Reagan. They were all over the country, and many of them were still living in Bloomfield, Michigan.

Easily, he won the election by beating the incumbent president by landslide. People were tired of the government, standing on the top of their heads and looking like the shape of a reversed pyramid. As soon as he took over the White House with the full support from his party and from the other side as well, he and his team wasted no time to make the government small and efficient by privatizing and downsizing government programs massively. He did not hesitate to push his agenda with full force. He started shutting down unnecessary government programs one by one or as many as he could.

Unfortunately, a lot of people, who had no idea or knowledge of this political turmoil, lost their job as a result of his budget cut. Young physicians who just got out of medical school were the first victims of Reagan's guillotine which the formerly failed movie actor brought into the White House.

This was why. This was what he did as a president. This was the first thing that he and his team did. He eliminated the budget for the residency training program of the entire country, with the exception of a few university hospitals, military hospitals, etc. As a matter of a fact, the government was paying the salary of the resident doctors of all the training hospitals. I have no idea how it started and which was the first one, whether the egg or the chicken. But most likely, the hospitals were unwilling or refused to invest the money for the training of the so-called specialists, and yet the society needed specialists so bad. So the government took care of the burden for the people. Quite naturally, in reality, it was the government that used to pay the salaries of the resident physicians, not the hospitals.

Mr. Reagan cut off the umbilical cord. Now it became the hospital's responsibility to pay the young doctors. Pay. Did I say "pay"? Hell no, no way. They did not pay. The hospitals did not pay, not even a single penny. How nice it was. The hospital hired the residents and made an enormous amount of money, but the government paid the salaries of the resident. What a country! So they turned around and eliminated the training program.

As a result of this budget cut, just in metropolitan Detroit only, hundreds of doctors in training lost their job. If we put all the numbers together with the entire fifty states, i.e., hundreds times fifty, the total number who lost their jobs would pile up like Mount Everest if we put one person on the top of another person and so on.

Think about it. Just imagine how much money the government saved as a result of eliminating this program only. I do not know anyone or do not have a friend working for the Congressional Budget Office. But the number would be staggering and still piling up even now and the future. Because the government will never bring back this program ever again. But it would be an enormous amount of money just to think about one year only or the next ten or twenty years and so on. The budget saves continues now and forever. Multiply the number of the residents who lost their jobs times their salaries and then times ten, twenty, or thirty years. I get headaches.

Only a few of the training hospitals that can afford to pay the residents was able to keep and maintain the resident training program. They survived and still produce specialists for the society. The government said, "If you can afford it, you can keep it. But if you cannot, too bad, we are not the answer to your problem anymore." Now does it sound familiar? The smell of capitalism? This was just only the beginning.

So many of government programs disappeared from our sight for good, and people loved it. Why? Mr. Reagan turned around our economy by sacrificing the few. States and cities copied the same.

Even the Democratic governors and mayors followed the same. Downsizing and privatizing became the bible of governing. Majority of the people were the beneficiaries of Mr. Reagan's policy.

By the way, who was the one person who got the most benefits from the economic turnaround by Mr. Reagan? It was—surprise—Mr. Bill Clinton. And you know the rest of the story.

Mr. Reagan will be remembered and respected by many, including myself, as a highly successful president who turned around our and the world economy from the bottom of the recession to a booming prosperity without the help of any war. Can you imagine that, as a person, he failed in his marriage and in his profession but, as a president, he became one of the top 3 most respected presidents in America's history? He is definitely one of the top 5, if not one of the top 3.

Then the question is what has anything to do with me and Mr. Reagan. Like anybody else, I was affected by his policy indirectly. By the way, tell me if there is anyone who felt no impact whatsoever by the sudden drastic change of his governing style? No sooner than Mr. Reagan and the Republicans eliminated the budget for the residency program that the hospital turned around and immediately started laying off the residents. They were pushed out to the street without knowing why.

The realty was when I became a second-year resident in internal medicine, half of my colleagues was gone. Gone with the wind. By the time I became a third-year resident, more than half of the remaining half was gone. In fact, only a few was left. But you were lucky if you were one of those few. In fact, I was the one of the few. Even now, I do not know how and why I survived.

Just imagine, the internal medicine department had usually more than ten third-year residents in the final year of the residency who were in charge of handling the entire hospital's inpatient and outpatient workload. And all of a sudden, a few was left, but the workloads were the same or increased. Not to mention about daytime work, but as far as night calls, when you become a third-year resident, you take three or four times a month in a usual scenario.

But the workload remained the same or worse because the number of my colleagues went down to less than a quarter, or worse, you have to take night calls once in three days, rather than three or four times a month.

America is such a huge country that it takes a long time for the people to feel the difference if or when Washington changes any law. By the time the general public feels the difference, those who made the changes, those who are responsible, are long gone. Whether you are going to be one of the victims or the beneficiaries, you never know what will happen to you, unless you are a Washington insider or you are the one who is making the changes.

So three years of training and the number of night calls did not change for me or got worse. And artificial insomnia, which was caused against my will and which I did not ask for, set in me permanently.

But again, I do not hate Mr. Reagan. As I mentioned earlier, I like him. Furthermore, I respect him. Because I know that he made all the changes not for himself but for the benefit of everybody, including myself, and even for Mr. Bill Clinton, who was the biggest beneficiary of Mr. Reagan's legacy. He did it for me, not for himself. When a politician does something for himself or a few of privileged ones, we the people suffer dearly. But when a politician does something for the people, we the people get the benefit ultimately.

Actually, the changes were coming everywhere. The changes were coming to the health insurance industry too. The concept of HMO (health maintenance organization) came in to play big role. I have to say this change was huge. It was unimaginable.

An insurance company hires a few doctors and nurses, and it decides whether not to pay or how much the health insurance is going to pay the hospitals and the doctors based on the diagnosis. Even how long a patient could have inpatient care was already determined by those few people who sat down in the well-air-conditioned office in hot summer weather. And the doctors have to discharge within a certain time frame, instead of out of necessity. Everything is dictated by the insurance. Even what kind of medicines the doctor can prescribe or not will be determined by the insurance company. The doctor has to choose among those medicines that the insurance company preselected. The government passed the law which allows the insurance company to come up with a tailor-made coverage based on the diagnosis rather than the patient's condition. The doctor or the hospital cannot keep the patient longer than the insurance company's mandate.

So when I graduated from the residency program and became a staff of doctor's group, the environment of medical practice changed drastically. Some days, I had to spend more time arguing with the insurance company on the phone, rather than taking care of my sick patients. After four years of practicing in the private sector and struggling with health insurance, I decided to move to something or somewhere else, choosing to join the hospital that belongs to the Michigan Department of Corrections.

It happened out of nowhere. It happened like this. On one afternoon, on a lunch break, my partner said, "Hey, do you want to go to Jackson?"

About forty minutes west of Ann Arbor in Jackson, Michigan, the biggest walled correctional facility in America is located. The biggest walled correctional facility in America means the biggest in the entire world. That's what the people who were working there said. They said, "Even the gate of heaven will open wide if you say you worked at the Jackson facility on earth. You do not need to worry about hell."

They are housing more than twenty thousand inmates and more than seven thousand correctional officers. In that facility, there is a small hospital called Duane L. Waters Hospital. It has one hundred inpatient beds, emergency room, operation rooms, laboratory, and radiology department as well. More than fifty doctors—surgeons, internists, psychiatrists, and dentists, and so on—are working in the hospital. So all the patients, including the terminally ill, come to Duane L. Waters Hospital to receive proper care by the doctor like me, until they go out healthy or they pass away.

I went to the hospital and was interviewed by the medical director, whose name by the way was Dr. Silas Norman and whose sister happened to be Jessye Norman, the world-famous classic opera singer. He himself was also an excellent classic baritone singer. At the end of the interview, he told me once I chose to work at the hospital and in case I decided to quit the next day due to whatever the reason it might be to come to his office exactly one year later and submit the letter of the resignation. He demanded, and I promised to do that. Because he already knew that I had heard all the scary things about inside the wall.

But somehow, immediately I began to like working for the prisoners—no, the inmates. They were like any other human beings. As I treated them and respected them, then they respected and treated me like any other human being. So I continued to work and treat sick people in the facility. One year became two, three, four, five, ten, almost twenty years. Professionally, those years were the best time of my entire life. Certainly, they were the golden days of my life.

It was one of those days. I forgot the date very soon, but you would find out why I remember the exact date if or when you finish reading this chapter. It was March 27, 1992, at lunch. After spending a busy morning as usual, I was enjoying my lunch with other staffs, correction officers, nurses, and secretaries in a small cafeteria on the first floor.

All of a sudden, I felt a sharp pain on the side of my rib cage. The nurse sitting next to me pinched or poked me without mercy. I do not remember how she did it, either with a fork or her long fingernail. She was pointing her finger at the correction officer, who was bending his neck and grabbing it with his both hands. I could not see his face but could see his earlobes whose color already turned almost black—maybe dark blue was the correct color—though he was a Caucasian man. As it turned out, he was a bit older than I was but was much bigger than I was.

Immediately, I recognized the situation. This was it! There was no time to think and no time to panic. Suddenly, there was no sound or no noise. There was nobody around. Just him and me. I found myself standing behind him. Then I helped him stand up. No, I put him up. His body felt like there were no bones or joints for me, and he was very heavy. He was a bit taller than I am. I am five feet ten or eleven inches tall. He was a bit over six feet. But he was a lot heavier than I was. He had a beard and a mustache and looked like big Santa. I tried to put my arms around him. It was not easy. Due to his weight, the gravity was pulling him down constantly, and I had to keep him straight up to apply the Heimlich maneuver. At last, the first abdominal thrust. I thought I did it real hard. But there was no response.

Here came the second attempt. I used all my reserved muscle strength since I was born. But I was holding a heavy body with no breathing, ready to go where he came from.

So I had to do it again, the third abdominal thrust. Just before the third trial, exactly half of a second like a lightning or an electric current, something passed through my brain. If I put in writing, it is as follows: "If he does not wake up after the third trial, if there is no response, that's the end." Two things went through my mind. It was a prayer or something. First, it was directed to God, who was watching from above at the time it happened. It was almost like a half prayer and half threat to him, whoever he is. "Please save this person. If not, he is going to die now. Then you are responsible! Not me." Actually, I was begging him. I was desperate. Second, "If he dies now, what kind of doctor am I going to be in front of all these people? I became a physician to save people's life. I spent all the money, time, and energy to be the one who saves people's life. I'm going to be a failure, and all the efforts will be wasted and going down the drain." To tell you the truth, it did not last more than half of one second.

Boom! I did the third attempt. I felt his weight became a little bit lighter. I put his body onto the floor and lay down next to him and looked at his face. It seemed like a human color, a living human color. I checked his pulse and respiration. He had a pulse and was breathing. A few minutes later, he opened his eyes and tried to sit up. We sat down on the table together and then we went back to our post as usual.

And then two or three months passed.

On one morning, there was a message that the administrator was looking for me. I went to see him in the afternoon. He said the warden was the one who wanted to see me. He had no idea why.

Next morning, I went to the warden's office. His office was located in the other building. As soon as I showed up, he jumped up from his big chair and offered his big hand with a big smile. And he said, "Thank you very much for saving my officer." He called his secretary to bring the Employee of the Month award and an envelope with some cash. I do not remember how much it was, but enough to have pizzas for lunches with my staffs. There was another page of statement explaining what happened.

"How did you know?" I asked.

He said, "I know everything what's happening here." And then he said no doctor had ever been given this award in the history of the Michigan's correction department. Probably, it was not going to happen in the future either, he said.

A few days later, I met the officer at the same place. And I asked him what happened. At the lunch table, he was about to finish his lunch. He was eating the dessert. A small piece of cookie went into his air pipe suddenly and unexpectedly. He tried desperately to bring it up on his own so that he would not ruin other people's lunch. Instead of coming out, the small piece went down farther, and he passed out. He said he did not remember how long he was out, but he suddenly saw a bright sunlight in his eyes.

Then he went back to his post. But he could not continue his duty because of splitting headaches. He went to his superior and asked his permission to leave early, who asked for the reason because he rarely left his post early, something that never happened before. He told his superior what happened at the lunch table. The story went up and up through the commanding channel and finally to the warden's office.

But three or four months later, a strange thing started happening and continued on and on to my body, to be exact, on my right shoulder. Initially, it happened only at night, an excruciating pain on my right shoulder, waking me up at night, once, twice, then many times. Then it occurred during the day. What was going on? What happened? The pain got worse and worse and became unbearable. Finally, I had to go. I had to go to the hospital to find the reason, hoping it was not something bad.

The doctor ordered an X-ray of my shoulder. He came to me with the X-ray results and also with an interesting look and said, "You have a separation of the right shoulder. Can you think of any reason why? Have you injured your right shoulder lately?"

My immediate response was no. The doctor gave me a pain medicine and told me to come back if the pain did not go away and that I might need surgery if the pain got worse.

On the way home in the car, out of nowhere, lightning hit me. Oh yes, I did something! It was something called the Heimlich maneuver. I remembered what I had done to my shoulder. Most likely, I pulled apart my shoulder during one of those abdominal thrusts. That's when something happened. At the same time when I was doing the third attempt, I also remembered that I threatened someone upstairs, who might have done something to my shoulder. The nasty pain lasted for more than several years. Then it disappeared without saying goodbye to me. One day, it was gone. Even though the pain was gone, the evidence is still there. The separation of my right shoulder still stays with me even now.

By the way, at the beginning of this chapter, I mentioned about which side I choose between the American Red Cross back blow method and the Heimlich maneuver. As you might have recognized already, I am on the side of Dr. Heimlich. The reason is that in a situation of desperation, when life and death is on the line, why would you waste the time blowing a victim's back and then going to the next step, which is Heimlich maneuver? Don't waste any time or thinking. Just go to the one that works, which both sides do not dispute. That's what I did. Opportunity is bald on the back. You can grab it only on the front. There is nothing to grab on the back. If you miss the front, there is no way you can grab the opportunity from behind. Once you miss it, there is no such thing called second chance. When we are dealing with human life, your life and my life, there is no second chance. We have only one chance.

This is how it is written on my Employee of the Month certificate:

Charles E. Egler Correctional Facility, Jackson, Michigan
Employee of the Month Award

JOHN G. CHUN, M. D.

for maintaining a high level of professionalism, dedication, and outstanding performance

Presented for the month of May 1992 as recommended by the Employee of the Month Committee at the facility.

There was a second page explaining what happened.

State of Michigan
Department of Corrections

Dr. John Chun
Duane L. Waters Hospital
Charles E. Egeler Correctional Facility
3855 Cooper Street Jackson, Michigan 49201

Re: Employee of the Month

Dear Dr. Chun:

I would like to take this opportunity to congratulate you on being chosen "Employee of the Month" for the Egeler Correctional Facility. Your action in applying the Heimlich maneuver to Officer Wayne [redacted] in the Duane Waters lunch room on March 27, 1992 showed quick thinking.

In fact, you may have saved Officer [redacted]'s life. Working for the Michigan Department of Correction is both a very difficult and demanding job. Professionalism of this type is both appreciated and respected.

On behalf of the entire staff at Egeler Facility, you are being congratulated for your fine service, and a job well done!

Sincerely,

Henry N. Grayson, Warden
Charles E. Egeler Correctional Facility

Because of this second page, I remember the date when it happened. Even if I forget the date and time again and again, I always can go back and pull out these two pages and remember and recall exactly how it happened.

It will be always with me, unless I develop something called memory loss, i.e., dementia. But the good news is that we can prevent dementia by keeping our blood pressure under control and with true exercise. I'll explain this good news in chapter 19, "Conclusion," briefly.

I cannot reveal the last name of the correction officer because I do not have his permission to do so.

CHAPTER 18

Las Vegas, the Sin City?

Why? Why the Sin City? Are the people living in Las Vegas all sinners or criminals just because they are living in Las Vegas? Of course not. Or do the people who went to Las Vegas for a nice vacation or business become sinners when they come back home? Certainly not. Neither is true.

Actually, the citizens of Las Vegas like to call their city "the entertainment capital of the world." But depending on what you do in Las Vegas with your hard-earned money, Vegas becomes the Sin City or the entertainment capital of the world. It is up to your behavior.

Living in Ann Arbor, Michigan, I like to go to Las Vegas in the winter. Winter only. Only in winter. You can stay in Michigan the rest of the year. If you enjoy winter weather and winter sports, you do not need to go anywhere else. Just stay in Michigan.

I do agree that the weather in winter season is particularly cruel in the northern parts of states, like Michigan, Minnesota, Wisconsin, New York, etc., not to mention Canada. So I'm one of the many who need to go to a warm place in winter, once or twice, the more, the better. Quite naturally, Las Vegas became one of my favorite destinations that I like to go in wintertime.

It became a lot better and warmer in winter in Michigan due to global warming compared to ten, twenty, thirty, or forty years ago. But by the time December comes, cold gets colder. I have to go somewhere, somewhere I can relax. I guess I'm one of those who suffer from a condition called cabin fever.

Generally, my favorite destination is Florida or Cancun, Mexico, in January when I need to melt down my frozen mind and Las Vegas in February when I need a little bit of entertainment along with warm weather.

When March is here, winter is gone in Michigan. Michigan has the best weather in spring, summer, and fall. You do not need to go anywhere during warm season. Do you remember that I traveled to Europe in late fall before winter came and in early spring just about when winter was over? During winter, it's time for Florida, Mexico, and especially Vegas.

Now I'm about to talk about Las Vegas. But to tell you the truth, although it is good place to have a fun, Vegas is not a good place to live. I have friends who moved to Las Vegas after retiring. But I have no intention to move to Vegas after my retirement.

As usual, let's talk about the bad news first. Is it not a good place to live? Two things come into my mind, weather and gambling. Maybe in terms of winter weather, Vegas has one of the best. However, for the rest of the year, remember where Vegas is located. Next to Mojave Desert and right next to Death Valley. And the entire city is filled with casinos. Is it not bad enough?

Next, let's talk about the good news! Can you think of any city better than Vegas in terms of entertainment? It has excellent scenery, good sightseeing, so many places to go, so many things to do, so many good places to eat, etc. It is the entertainment capital of the world. I agree 100 percent.

Let's talk about gambling, i.e., casinos. Recently, in the USA, casinos popped up everywhere; big city or small city, it doesn't matter. It is a worrisome reality, but instead of worrying, it's time to find a solution on our own. In the past, it was watching fire across the street or across the river. Now it became fire on my shoes. In the past, in order to go to a casino, we had to go to Las Vegas or Atlantic City, which means we had to go there by air. Now if we want to go to a casino, we can drive for less than an hour in any direction.

Why? By whom? First, by whom? By politician is the answer. And why? In American politics, there is one thing politicians should never say, even while in their sleep. It is tax. Never talk about raising tax, no matter how good your intention might be and no matter how bad the economy might be. No matter how bad the economy may be, if the politician mentions about tax hike to solve the problem, the moment they say it, they are dead politically. Even if they got elected, they should never talk about increasing taxes. During the campaign for the second term, wherever he went, one-term president Father Bush said to the audience, pointing his lips, "Read my lips. No new taxes." But he increased tax as soon as he became the president. That was his fatal mistake for his second-term election.

So we don't know whose idea it was and where it came from, casino became the solution. By taking advantage of the gambling "gene" that we all have, billionaires, not millionaires, will collect money with ease from the average person like you or me. And politicians collect tax from casinos. They don't have to increase tax. It is just a matter of time for the average Joe to go bankrupt by gambling.

As a result, casinos are popping up everywhere. Here in Ann Arbor, it takes only thirty or forty minutes to go to downtown Detroit where three big casinos are enjoying booming business. From downtown Detroit to Windsor, Canada, taking only ten minutes or so, we can reach one of the biggest casinos in Canada. From Ann Arbor to Toledo, Ohio, taking thirty to forty minutes, there is another huge casino. From Ann Arbor to the west on the way to Chicago, about one hour distance, another casino is waiting for the average Joe. Open for twenty-four hours, day and night, they are waiting. Who cares whether we would go bankrupt or not? No one cares.

It is something that we did not witness before. It is becoming a social issue. No, it became a social issue already. I'm concerned about drug addiction, alcohol addiction, nicotine addiction, food addiction, and gambling addiction. I worry about the future of America. I worry about my future and my future generations and so on. Among addictions, we can think about the following five: alcohol, nicotine, drugs, food, and, last but not the least, gambling.

I'm going to talk about why we shouldn't go to Vegas first and then why we should go next.

Before gambling, let's talk about alcoholism. Generally, there are three different groups of people. First, the people who were born with a sufficient number of alcoholic gene. So no matter how much and what kind of alcohol they may drink, it doesn't bother them. We call them Superman or Wonder Woman. But at the end, ultimately they ruin not only their body but also their mind and not only themselves but also their innocent family. Then we call them alcoholics. Second, the people who were born with no or almost no alcoholic gene so that their faces turn red even with the smell of alcohol. Third, the people in the middle, who are more than the second group but a lot less than the first. So that if these people happened to be surrounded by the first group, quite naturally and eventually, they become alcoholic. If surrounded by the second group of people, they remain and belong to the second group.

The definition of alcoholism has nothing to do with the amount of alcohol one is able to drink. The definition of alcoholism is as follows: "any drinking of alcohol that results in problem." If drinking alcohol causes any problem to you, to your family, to your job, and ultimately to the society, you are an alcoholic. It does not matter how much you drink or how strong the alcohol is. If you cannot be on time in your class or in your cubicle the next morning after drinking the night before, sorry, you are an alcoholic. You have an alcohol addiction. If you have a problem, your family and the society would also have a problem.

But if there is something that worries me the most—I have to say the worst—it is gun violence or gun addiction in America. I grew up in a country where no gun is visible, i.e., available. I never saw a gun or even a hunting rifle in my entire life, until in my late twenties when I came to the country of my dream called USA. I have to say it is everywhere. I can see it in the hunting or sporting goods section at Kmart, my favorite shopping store when I came to America forty years ago.

I was born in 1949, and the Korean War broke in 1950 and lasted three full years. By the time the war was over, I was too young to remember what was happening in terms of gun violence in Korea. But it must have been pretty bad.

By the time I was old enough to figure out what was going on, gun ownership was already illegal. The government acted pretty quick and efficiently because the gun violence was bad, real bad, immediately after the war. It was illegal for anyone to own a gun or any firearm. You had to have a license even to own a hunting rifle, and yet you had to keep the firearm at a police station and had to have the gun signed out and returned when you finished hunting. You could not keep it at home.

It is unimaginable if you are told that there are only a few deaths by gunshot from both homicide and suicide combined in a country with an entire population of fifty million people, one or two a year, sometimes none. Can you imagine a population of fifty million people has almost no gun-related death?

Living in a country named Korea for thirty years of my life since I was born until I came to a country called America, I've never heard any news from TV or newspaper that someone died by a gunshot wound.

What a waste of human lives. Just think that there are more than three hundred precious human lives a year lost in the city of Detroit only, with a population of less than a million. One precious life a day versus a few to none a year on the other side of this continent.

I grew up in a culture where and if there is any dispute or difference in opinion, we settle it with a fist or two, usually two because we needed both when we fight. Usually, we choose a very quiet place, such as a remote corner of a schoolyard with no audience. We do not need onlookers. Just between him and me. No one knows the result. It does not matter who won or who lost. It is top secret between him and me. The only reality between him and me is the fact that we became best friends after the fight. It does not matter what's the result, but we became best friends. We talk. We continue to talk to each other as best friends.

Here in America, if we have a dispute, it does not matter how old or young or whether male or female, usually male. Solving the dispute is very simple and short. All you need is a gun and an index finger. It does not matter whether there are any people around. And you do not need a schoolyard. It is just like Old Wild West. There is no talking. We cannot talk to each other if there is only one left, one left with a gun, and the other is gone with a hole or holes somewhere in the body. There are only two—the quick and the dead, sometimes only the quick and the many dead. There is no talking. You cannot talk to each other if there is only one left, left in jail for the rest of his life. One or more than one are buried, and the one left will be in jail for life.

I'm going to end the discussion of this particular issue, leaving it to difference of opinion. Do you remember that we agree to disagree? Especially because this book is a book of life and is about how to live long and healthy.

Let us go back to gambling, as in alcoholism. First, the people who were born with a sufficient number of gambling gene are living with a high probability to get addicted, and once exposed, there is a high chance they would ruin not only their life but also their family's. Second, the people who were born with no gambling gene or almost no gambling gene are living their entire life without the urge to go to a casino. This people have no chance or almost no chance to get addicted. Third, the people who are in the middle, who have more gambling genes than the second group but a lot less than the first. So that if these people, the third group, happened to be surrounded by the first group, they remain and belong to the first group. But if these people happened to be surrounded by the second group, they will belong and remain in the second group.

I sincerely hope and pray for the people in the third group and second group as well. But there is only one exception.

You are retired, and all the retirement plans are in place. You are old and accomplished. Why not give all your assets to your next generation already? And then with your leftover, enjoy your life, whichever way you choose. Gambling is good for the prevention of dementia, some say. But if you have dementia already, hopefully you forgot about gambling as well. The following are the reasons why we shouldn't gamble.

One, there is no chance and no probability. Especially the chance goes low and low if you stay longer. The longer you stay, the less your chance is going to be. Why do you start a war when your chance of winning is so low that even you know you are going to lose? Because it is fun? What kind of fun is that? Are you having fun losing your hard-earned money? Nonsense!

We have no chance with a table game. The longer you sit there, for sure the less your chance will be. You have to decide whether to stay or fold before the dealer. What a disadvantage it is! What a nonsense. Statistically, the chance to lose or win is between 49 percent to 51 percent. It's pretty high, but do not be fooled by the numbers.

And in slot machine, it is worse, much worse than the table game. Here's a personal story I heard from a taxi driver. For more than ten years, he worked hard day and night as a dealer to save enough money to own and run a small business. When he said to himself that the time had come, he decided to go to the casino where he used to work as a customer, not as a dealer, just for one day, only one day. That one day became two days, then three days, and so on. All his money were gone, and he could not leave Vegas, and he became a taxi driver.

Again we, average Joes, lose again. This time, it is a psychological warfare. The geniuses in math and psychology who graduated from the Ivy League, Big Ten Conference, and Pac-12 Conference are working for casinos behind the curtain. We, the average Joes, are no match for those geniuses. Give up to win in casino against these people, the geniuses. You and I are no match against them.

Here are the three no's in casino:

* No window to look outside. We cannot see outside and, hence, cannot see reality. There is no chance to other people, other than the gambler like yourself. There is no chance to see the reality outside. "Why I'm here? What am I doing here? Why I'm not there?" You have no chance to ask these questions.
* No mirrors around you, except when you are in the restrooms. You cannot see your face while gambling. You cannot see your face, the face of a loser.
* No clocks on the wall. Unless you have your own watch, you cannot tell or see whether the sun is out or the moon is out.

So once you step in a casino, you lose the concept of time, numbers, reality, and so on. Especially you lose the concept of money.

The value of money disappears. Like someone who goes to grocery stores or department stores and looks for items that are one dollar cheaper but suddenly throws away a one-hundred-dollar bill on the table like it is a one-dollar bill.

In the whole USA, no one can smoke inside any of the public places, but there is only one exception. That is casinos. You can smoke in casinos in the USA, but not in Canada.

When I go to Vegas, I see someone that I know who moved to Vegas from Michigan. They say Vegas is so good that they highly recommend anybody to move to Vegas after retiring. They say it was the best decision that they have ever made. But they never fail to mention at the end that Vegas will be your dream come true only if you have the willpower to stay away from casinos. So throw away your greed and open the window of your mind. Then something good will fly into your mind.

Now let's talk about the reason we have to go to Vegas. For your own information, here is a list of places that people want to go to on a winter vacation. The public poll shows number 1, Las Vegas; number 2, Cancun, Mexico; and number 3, Orlando, Florida, where Disney World is located.

First, even though part of the reason I do not recommend moving to Vegas after retirement is due to the hot summer weather, where in the world can you find a better place for entertainment for the winter vacation? I have never been to Las Vegas in summertime so far. So I cannot comment about the summer weather in Vegas. Again, Death Valley is only two hours away from Vegas. That's all I can say. Anyway, if you go to Vegas in winter, the weather feels like late autumn. When the sun is out, it is warm. But when the sun goes down, it is quite chilly. That is all for the weather.

Second, to attract casino customers, the other expenses are relatively cheaper than you think—prices of hotel, airplane, food, etc. There are many excellent shows and performances everywhere. Talking about food, the city has the top 10 buffet restaurants in the whole USA. When we say the city is the entertainment capital of the world, it also includes entertaining our taste buds.

Third, you can go to the Grand Canyon and the Hoover Dam. One is God made; the other is man-made. How magnificent these two are. I'm not going to describe the Grand Canyon or the Hoover Dam here because it's impossible. It is as simple as that. It is impossible. You have to see it to believe it and agree with my point. People are coming all over the world. Tourists are coming to Las Vegas to see the Grand Canyon.

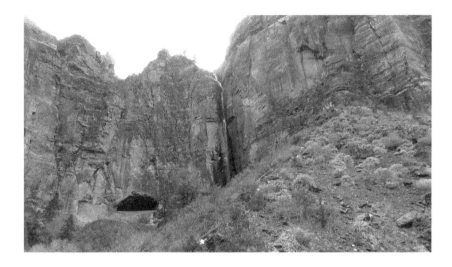

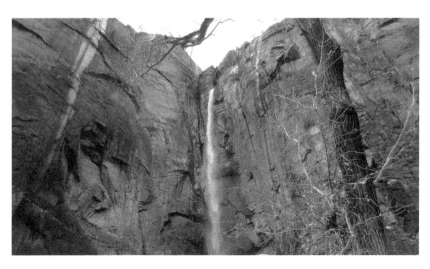

Fourth, if you drive to the direction of Utah, in about two and half hours, you will meet Zion National Park and, in about four hours, Bryce Canyon National Park. Again, I'm not going to describe about how magnificent they are. But especially when you go to Zion National Park, you wouldn't want to come home. You would want to stay there for good.

Fifth, there are many good golf courses around the city. Golf is an excellent tool to stay away from gambling.

Sixth, there are excellent shows and performances in the evening.

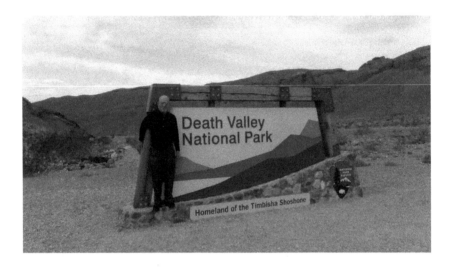

Seventh, two hours from Vegas toward California, you can visit Death Valley. If you have not been to this one, I highly recommend to visit the amazing national park once. It is up to you to go again whenever you go to Las Vegas, like me. Go to the bottom of the big valley. And then go to the top and see the valley.

If you are involved in all these activities, you would not have much time to sit on the gambling table. Make yourself busy and stay away from the casinos. Spend more time outside. Believe it or not.

A long, long time ago, there was a very rich man. When he was about to die, he prayed to God if he could carry his hard-earned fortune into the afterlife. His prayer was so intense that God could not refuse. He got the permission from God. With all his money, he bought gold, thinking that only gold is accepted in heaven. Finally, when he died, he entered the gate of heaven, with his gold on his back, sweating all over his body. Upon his arrival, the people in heaven were whispering, "We have gold everywhere here, and everything is free. Why does he have to sweat for gold?" Indeed, he saw gold everywhere in heaven. In buildings, streets, everywhere, he saw gold. And everything was free.

We do not need money or gold in heaven. When we go to heaven, leave everything behind and then go empty-handed.

At the moment we came to this world, we are screaming as hard as we can, as if somebody beat our behind real bad. We make our fist as hard as we can, as if we have something precious in our hands, although we had nothing in our hands, or as if we are a boxer ready to fight. But when we are ready to go back to where we came from, we close our eyes softly so that we can open our eyes any time to see God any moment. We keep our hands empty so that we can grab his hands strongly with our two hands. If we are holding something already in our hands, how can we grab his hands? Humbly, we put our hands on the belly so that we can grab his hands real quick and hard rather than in the back. How can he grab our hands if we are hiding our hands on the back? And our two ears are wide open and our mouth is shut so that we are ready to hear anything since we are done talking. This is the way we are when we go back to where we came from.

CHAPTER 19

Conclusion

As I mentioned at the beginning of this book, I already discussed the conclusions and the solutions of each health-related chapter. I have absolutely no intention to waste your precious time and mine as well just to repeat what I said already. Heck no! Instead, I'm going to discuss about the two most important issues of our lives.

The first and the most important of all is how to go back to where we all came from. And the second most important one is how to deal with the seven most evil malfunctions of our body. Each one of them has to be dealt with the most advanced scientific way and has to be defeated soundly in the most efficient way.

I already talked about how to be healthy and live long throughout this book. At the end of each health-related chapter, I gave you the solutions, i.e., how to achieve the goal.

First, let me talk about the seven evils. I'm going to finish my book talking about seven most common reasons that can easily jeopardize our quality of life, which I call seven evils. I'd like to avoid these seven evils at all costs. Of course, prevention is very important. But if and when something evil comes into our body, then we have no choice but to fight back and defeat the evils. This is how to defeat those seven evils. Then what are they?

1. hypertension
2. heart attack

3. stroke
4. dementia
5. cancer
6. diabetes
7. car accident

These are my concerns. I'm sure these are your concerns too. When something bad happens in our lives, it happens. No matter how you want to avoid these evils, it happens when it happens. Sometimes, we have no choice. Let's say, if you were born with this evil printed on your DNA, you cannot avoid this but to fight and defeat and win. In this situation, we can say, "To be or not to be."

Yes, if you do what I'm telling you to do, the outcome of those bad things will be drastically different. This is how to deal with the seven evils.

Can we defeat these seven evils? The answer is yes, we can. Are there ways to avoid these seven? The answer is yes, there are.

But unfortunately, hypertension belongs to one of the seven evils and might be or could be the underlying cause of the other three. More than half of the seven evils are related with hypertension.

This is what I will do to maintain my health. I try everything that I can. Then I pray. But I do know there are many people who do not try or barely try their best and who just pray. Please do your best first, then pray. Or at least, do both at the same time. I hope there are less people in the second group than I think. I hope everyone belongs to my group. Long before me, someone said already, "Heaven helps those who help themselves." We all should belong to this group. We have to do our best and then pray. We have to do our best and then ask for miracle and/or our Father's mercy.

This is how to deal with the seven evils.

Number 1: hypertension

I hope or wish this one does not occur to you and me. Sincerely, I pray that this evil does not occur to us. But unfortunately, with time, this evil will occur to all of us or most of us, no matter what we do and no matter how hard we pray. We cannot avoid this evil. With age, as we grow older, most of us, if not all, will have to face this evil one way or another, genetically or environmentally. Do you remember degenerative changes, i.e., aging process, and vice versa? It is just a matter of when, how soon, or how late. It is inevitable.

We have to face it and fight to win. We all go through these degenerative changes because our blood vessels, particularly arteries, will lose their God-given flexibility, i.e., elasticity, as we grow older, with no exception. The blood pressure will go up slowly but surely or sometimes suddenly, with no warnings whatsoever, with little or no symptom at all. It will cause serious damage to our vital organs and make our lives as miserable as it can. That is why it is called the "silent killer."

But first thing first. Who is responsible to find or pick up this monster? Is it your doctor or nurse? Definitely it is not them. Then who? And how do we find it when I said there is little or no symptom?

It is you or me. We have to find our own monster hiding inside our body with a small equipment called blood pressure cuff, which you can buy at any other drugstore or Costco at a reasonable price. The sooner, the better. If your blood pressure is mildly elevated, you can control this monster without taking medicine. Remember exercise? Diet? Combination of both? Yes, it is your duty to pick up your high blood pressure. Then it's your doctor's turn and his duty to treat your hypertension. Again, it's our duty to find it, and it's the doctor's duty to treat it.

Long time ago when I was an intern, there was only a few medicines available for this condition with serious side effects. Now in the modern days of the twenty-first century, we have more than enough of blood pressure medicines with less side effects. Your doctor needs to find one or two, if necessary, to fit your condition.

So when and if your blood pressure goes up, please do not deny nature or the truth. Accept the fact and the truth as it is. Do not waste your valuable time. Your only choice is to take action immediately—meaning, find a good doctor and start taking proper medicine.

Now the choice is yours. Before you pray, please change your lifestyle, take appropriate medicine, and change your eating habit for the better. If you are doing something bad for your health—such as smoking, drinking alcohol excessively, etc.—then quit. You have no choice. If you are doing good for your health—such as exercising constantly, sleeping well, and drinking water wisely, etc.—then continue.

Now this is as summary of how to defeat hypertension, the silent killer:

1.   Change your lifestyle and eating habit for the better.
2.   Detect your elevated blood pressure as early as possible and go to your good doctor who will find a good medicine for you. And take the medicine religiously.
3.   Exercise and then pray.

Number 2: heart attack

I hope and pray this nasty and evil event does not occur to you and me. Again, before we pray, we have to do certain things if we want to avoid or defeat this evil.

Yes, when it happens, it happens. But we can prevent this before it happens if we do certain things, such as controlling blood pressure, taking aspirin, and doing exercise, etc. Yes, we can prevent this if we do what I'm telling us to do now. We can defeat this evil if we detect it early and take a proper medicine

There are two most common reasons when the coronary arteries supplying oxygens and nutrition to the heart muscles fail to perform its function, which are blockage and rupture of the vessels.

For the blockage, there are two reasons. One is the blockage that developed at the site of blockage, i.e., thrombus formation. And the other is the one that originated and came from other parts of our body, i.e., embolism or embolus. To minimize or prevent this evil event, for prophylaxis, we must take aspirin and do true exercise as well as other nonmedical measures.

For the rupture, it is more difficult to explain than thrombus or embolism. It is a bit complicated. A rupture of blood vessel happens at the coronary arteries that supply the heart muscles. When we talk about rupture of blood vessels, it is usually or almost always rupture of aneurysm that occurs at a certain part of blood vessels. When it happens at a big vessel, it's a big heart attack, and when it happens at a small blood vessel, a small heart attack. This process also applies to stroke. An aneurysm is a small balloonlike structure with thin and weakened wall anywhere in the arterial system, usually or almost always caused by a high pressure inside the vessel, which is hypertension. Normally, when the heart is relaxing (diastolic phase), the pressure inside the arteries remains somewhere around 80 mm Hg. And when the heart is squeezing or contracting (systolic phase), the pressure inside goes up to 120 mm Hg. This is our normal blood pressure of 120/80 mm Hg.

Whatever the reason is, when the pressure goes up, we call it hypertension, which is the most common cause of an aneurysm. When it bursts in our heart, we call it a heart attack. And when it happens in our brain, we call it a stroke.

So when the time comes, the wall of aneurysm becomes so thin that it ruptures with even a slight increase of the pressure inside, with no reason whatsoever or with no warning whatsoever. To minimize or prevent this particular event, as prophylaxis, we must do the best we can to control our blood pressure at all costs.

Now the choice is yours. Yes, you have to pray. But we have to put more effort to control the monster. Before you pray, change your lifestyle and eating habit. If you are doing bad things for your health, stop it. If you are not doing something good for health, then find something good because you know what those are. Go back and read the six elements of good health and hypertension.

Now in summary, this is what we have to do to prevent heart attack:

1. Change your lifestyle and eating habit. Talk to your doctor and take their advices.
2. Take one baby aspirin a day, unless you have any reason not to take or you are already taking nonsteroidal antiinflammatory drugs, such as Motrin, etc.
3. Read "Number 1: hypertension."
4. Exercise and then pray.

Number 3: stroke

It is kind of easier to explain the mechanism and the cause of this evil after I explained about heart attack and hypertension already. The most common cause of stroke is almost the same as in heart attack. Something real bad happens at blood vessels in the brain, such as thrombus, embolism, aneurysm, and so on. On top of all the above, please do not forget the aging process, i.e., degenerative changes, that happens in our entire body.

At the same time, our blood pressure fluctuates, and you never know when it happens. If it happens at big vessels, it will be a big stroke. Luckily, if it happens at small vessels, it will be a small stroke. But do not wait until it happens to you. Do something before a bad thing happens to you. Like any other disasters, early detection and prevention before something bad happens will be the best remedy that we can do for ourselves. We call this evil an "accident" that happens in our brain. Yes, accident does happen in our lives, but we have to do everything and anything to prevent this evil at all costs. Consider the financial loss and emotional damage before and after the accident, which can cripple not only you but also your entire family.

So this is how we fight and defeat this evil:

1. Change your lifestyle and eating habit.
2. Take one baby aspirin a day if you do not have any contra-indication to take it.
3. Control your high blood pressure before it's too late.
4. Go back and read "Number 1: hypertension" and "Number 2: heart attack."
5. Exercise and don't forget to pray.

Number 4: dementia

I hope and wish this one does not occur to you and me. But it breaks my heart that too many people around us are suffering from this one. It was a very rare disease that only a few or not so many people were suffering in the entire village where I grew up. Now it is everywhere. Are we living too long?

It makes me sad that when I go to my refrigerator, I forgot why I went there. Is it one of normal forgetfulness with normal aging process or an early sign of something evil whose name starts with D?

I'm not going to waste our time talking about a rare genetic disease causing dementia. There are many different causes of dementia. But I'm going to discuss about the most common cause of dementia called vascular dementia, which is related with blood vessels. Sounds familiar? Yes, it is caused by a certain change in small almost-invisible blood vessels called capillaries, associated with elevated blood pressure, combined with degenerative changes, i.e., aging process.

Again, do not wait until it happens to you. Because it is too late by the time this evil shows up in front of your door. There is no turning back. We have to prevent this evil before it knocks on the front door. Of course, we cannot prevent the degenerative changes. But definitely, we can prevent and defeat high blood pressure and, as a result of it, dementia as well.

So if and when we control blood pressure, we defeat how many evils? Not just one or two, we can defeat three more evils. Altogether, we defeat four of them—hypertension, heart attack, stroke, and dementia.

Let me explain to you how vascular dementia occurs in our brain as simple as I can. Let's suppose there is someone who has had high blood pressure at a young age that is left untreated for a long time. Then what happens to their brain?

From time to time, a small capillary on the arterial side of the brain will suffer from microscopic hemorrhages after hemorrhages over a long time. It bursts, and healing repeats itself over and over again. They might feel a slight headache or no headache at all. This is what happens at the vascular or capillary level. Then what happens at the tissue level? What happens to our brain tissue itself? Due to—complete at worst or partial at best—lack of oxygen and nutrition, our valuable brain tissue dies. If this person's hypertension is left untreated for ten, twenty, or thirty years, the vicious cycle will repeat and repeat and repeat, until the normal tissues are replaced by scar tissues, where there is no normal function to be seen. Once normal tissues are replaced by scar tissues, there is no turning back. Have you ever seen a scar tissue on the skin going back to normal skin? It will never go back to normal skin. The same thing will happen inside our brain.

Then what happens? We will forget small things, then big things. We will forget recent memories, then remote memories. We will forget what our iPhone does for us. The iPhone becomes meaningless because we do not recognize what it is. I'm going to stop here about the clinical manifestations of dementia. It is depressing. Let's move to how to prevent this monster.

The truth is once it happens, there is no cure for this evil. We cannot turn back time. All we can do is prevention. Detect on time and do something before it's too late. We have to do something before this evil occurs to us. Do you remember hypertension?

So what do we have to do? The answer is very simple. You should not miss what I'm about to say. Please remember that prevention is the key. This is how to prevent dementia. This is how to defeat dementia.

1. Buy a blood pressure cuff, search, and kill. No, search and treat at all costs if your blood pressure is high. Always remember the cost before and after.
2. Change your lifestyle and eating habits.
3. Go back and read "Number 1: hypertension" again.
4. Exercise and then pray.

Number 5: cancer

I hope and pray this evil does not occur to you and me. But sometimes, a bad thing happens, and we have no choice but to face it and fight. We have to pass through it. We cannot and will not bypass it once it happens.

When you are told that you have this evil inside your body, the situation is entirely different in the twenty-first century than in the twentieth century when I just got out of my medical school.

Yes, you are disappointed and even depressed. You have every right to get depressed. But make it short. The lesser and the shorter, the better this time. And then you have to stand up and fight this enemy. This could be the worst nightmare that you have ever faced all your life. You can get depressed for a while but don't take too long. This could be the worst challenge of your lifetime, whose outcome might be totally dependent on someone called an oncologist because a doctor-patient relationship is such an important factor in cancer treatment. We are very fortunate that we are living in a country called America, where we can receive the best state-of-the-art therapy we cannot imagine anywhere in this world.

Now we are living in a world where and a time when cancer is no longer untreatable or unbeatable, except in a few instances. We can go back to where you were and become cancer-free like you used to. America has the best health care system. And trust the system and the doctors, especially the oncologists, and listen to them and follow whatever they say. They are the best. Why? Because I say so.

The treatment of cancer has advanced so drastically compared to twenty, ten, or even one year ago. And new studies and new treatment methods of chemotherapy, radiation therapy, and especially immunotherapy, utilizing our own T cells—which not only can kill cancer cells selectively but also can remove the mutated part of DNA, which is responsible for the cancer, which scientists call "scissors"—available for many different cancers are coming out monthly, weekly, and almost daily even.

Just be patient. It is only a matter of short time that modern medicine comes up with the cure for the cancers. Or the good news is that it is just a few steps away from us. Maybe the sun is already on the horizon. And it is time for it to shine above us. So do not give up. And look around us. There are so many people proudly claiming themselves cancer-free or cancer survivors. There are many.

I do not need to emphasize how important early detection is in cancer treatment.

Before I finish this section, I have to remind you about something. Do you remember what I said earlier about the relationship between alkalosis and cancer, i.e., exercise and cancer? Cancer hates alkalosis. Am I too optimistic? Or realistic?

So I do not need to repeat how to defeat cancer. Read this chapter carefully. And then exercise and pray all the time.

Number 6: diabetes

I hope and wish this annoying headache does not occur to you and me. But it is almost impossible to avoid this evil if we consider and compare the enormous amount of food, i.e., calories, we put into our body, not to mention the quality itself and the amount of exercise we do.

At around the middle age of forties and fifties, we all go through the aging process and begin to suffer from one or more than one of metabolic syndromes, such as high blood pressure, high cholesterol, high blood sugar, and early signs of arthritis, etc.

Like blood pressure, when our blood sugar goes up, we do not feel anything. There is no warning sign whatsoever. If you are a very sensitive person, you might feel easily getting tired and/or losing or gaining weight excessively and might realize three important symptoms and signs later, such as eating a lot, drinking water a lot, and peeing a lot. We call this adult-onset diabetes mellitus or type 2 diabetes mellitus as opposed to juvenile-onset diabetes mellitus or type 1 diabetes mellitus.

Here, I'm talking about type 2 diabetes mellitus, which happens mostly after we became an adult and hence is associated with aging. Again, when it happens, it happens. As I mentioned before, like hypertension, it was a big deal forty or fifty years ago because we did not have good weapons to fight and defeat this disease. But not anymore. Guess what? We have enough or more than enough weapons to fight this disease.

With the above symptoms and signs and with diagnostic testing, you can confirm the diagnosis with the help of your good doctor. Receive a good medicine or two among those many antidiabetic agents.

But there is good news. As in hypertension, we can treat this evil without taking medicine if your blood sugar is not highly or mildly elevated. Do you remember exercise? Exercise can burn unnecessary blood sugar and bring it down to normal or close to normal.

So this is how to defeat this evil:

1. Change your lifestyle and eating habit. You might need to see a dietitian if necessary.
2. Take a medicine or two if necessary, sometimes insulin shots. But most type 2s can be controlled with pills and exercise.
3. Do not forget to exercise.
4. Is it necessary to pray? God is busy. And his Son too.

Number 7: car accident

I hope and pray this evil does not happen to you and me. But sometimes or many times, this happens when it happens, without warning or no matter how careful you might be. You have done everything I said and are in good health physically and mentally. You are in perfect condition as anyone wants to be. But accidents do occur by me or by others too.

For example, a car accident that is caused by you is very unfortunate. But if you want to prevent this tragedy from happening in the future, all you can do is be more careful and pray more or better. If you are not careful, there is no reason to pray. Why bother?

A car accident that is caused by others—for example, by a young person who was sending text messages to her boyfriend or to his girlfriend while driving—I have no comment for you. It is not your fault; it is 100 percent someone else's fault. Unfortunately, there is no way you can prevent this tragedy. When you are walking with your friend in a busy street, a brick on the roof of a building got loose and fell to the ground, but the brick hit the top of your head before hitting the ground. It is 100 percent not your fault. There is no way you can prevent this kind of accidents.

But theoretically, if you are very careful, such as driving within the speed limit and keeping a safe distance from the car in front of you, and pray good enough, you can prevent 50 percent of all accidents that could happen to you.

Before I move on to the next subject, I have to make it clear that simply because I said to pray at the end does not mean that we pray only at the end. Actually, we have to pray all the time, but the priority is we have to do our best while praying. I'm emphasizing that doing our best is also important.

As a matter of fact, the main subject of this book is health. When I'm talking about health-related subjects, I always put the conclusion, i.e., the solution, at the end of each chapter. I did not invent these solutions. To be honest, they were invented by someone else. All I have done is put one thing or two together—exactly speaking, six—to work for our body to live long and healthy.

Again, the solution for good health is exercise. Exercise, exercise, and exercise. And work out, work out, and work out. It does not matter how old you are. It does not matter whether you are female or male. Even if you are paralyzed on a certain part of your body, you have to exercise those other parts of your body that you can move. Exercise is an essential, not a luxury. Exercise is something that you have to do. It is not something that you do if you can or something you do not do if you cannot.

You do not have to do stairs exercise, which I recommend the most. You do not have to do it only because I recommend. If you have your own way of exercising, that is all I'm asking. It does not matter, as long as it fits the definition of true exercise. If it fits your particular condition or your ability or you can develop a certain exercise that fits just for you, then that is the best exercise for you. If you have your kind of exercise already, I recommend you continue your exercise and add one of those that I recommended. It does not matter if the methods are different, as long as we reach the same goal. It is important to arrive at the same finish line and cut the tape with our big chest and strong muscular lower extremities. The finish line, the goal of each exercise, is to give our body the gift of respiratory alkalosis and endorphin.

We humans are very unique and mysterious creatures that we have to do exercise all the time. We even did exercise before we were born. Sometimes, we kicked our mamas' sides so hard that our mamas had to wake up in the middle of the night. And we were swimming before we were born. If you look at newborn babies, they exercise all the time, except when they are sleeping.

We like to watch those athletes whom we like. When my favorite Tigers hits a home run, I feel like I did it. Almost, I confuse myself with the athlete I like. That's how much we like to exercise.

So I put all the solutions together in one sentence again: The path to good health should be a combination of proper exercising, drinking water wisely, and sleeping well. And then keep your oral hygiene decent while you take aspirin and Pepcid once a day.

I came up with and created a formula combining all the above six elements:

formula 1: good health = exercise + water + sleep + baby aspirin + acid controller + oral hygiene

Out of the six elements of good health, exercise will provide us with two of the most fascinating gifts of our lives, which seem to come down from heaven. First, during the vigorous muscle activities, exercise will stimulate our two lungs and help our body transform from an acidotic to an alkalotic environment. Second, when our body becomes alkalotic, it will trigger the pituitary gland, the control center of all hormones, to produce endorphins. In return, these two products, generated by true exercise, will give us fourteen of what I call small miracles described in the chapter "Exercise, the Most Important of All."

Then there is formula 2:

true exercise = respiratory alkalosis + endorphin (which produce small miracles of fourteen)

Work hard on what you do every day and save enough money for your hobby. Hopefully, it's traveling. And enjoy traveling. I recommend traveling. Traveling overseas—just thinking about it makes me get excited. I have three places to recommend, maybe four: Rome, Alaska, Barcelona, and Egypt.

Once is not enough; twice is not enough and so on. Like old friends who grew up together and who do not need to talk, just looking at each other is more than enough. The meeting could be their last, but they are still promising each other to meet again like old friends.

First, easy one: Barcelona, Spain.

I recommend a group tour. This is not a small country located in the east end of Europe, along with Portugal. When you go to Spain, always include Madrid and Barcelona. If you are a Catholic, make sure to visit Montserrat, an hour from Barcelona. Also make sure you have enough time to meet the Black Madonna.

Rome

It is the best place to travel alone or with just a few good friends or two couples after you had a chance or two to get familiarized with each other—you and Rome. I have seen many solitary travelers.

If you research about the history of Italy, then you will learn a lot more after each travel, which would make you want to go Rome over and over again. In fact, it is a very safe place to travel in Europe, especially Rome, Italy. You do not have to worry about safety.

When you go to Rome alone or with a few, utilize public transportation, especially bus. Because you can see outside in the bus. Another thing that you must not forget is that the hotel you are staying in should be close to a terminal.

When you go to Rome, include another place or city of a different variety, such as Milano, Venice, Florence, Santa Lucia, etc.

Alaska

I recommend solo traveling or with a few. Unlike any other traveling, you need peace and quiet. Two couples would be ideal. Sometimes, you have to choose either being in a group or with an entire family traveling together, like a cruise. Other than on special occasions, if you want to mix with nature and become one with it, I highly recommend you travel Alaska alone or with just a few.

Alaska is closest to the continent of US among those places I recommended. Go to Anchorage first and rent a car, an SUV, a minivan, or an RV, etc., at the airport—whatever you want—and go wherever you want. As far as I know, the Alaska airport is the only one where you can rent an RV.

You must include Denali in your Alaska trip. I mean Denali National Park. As you studied before you start, drive wherever the GPS tells you to go.

Egypt

You have to travel in a group from the beginning. You have to consider your safety also.

Like any other travel, you have to study real hard about the history of ancient Egypt if you want to make the most out of this particular travel. You have to choose a travel package which includes Nile river cruise and Abu Simbel and spend at least two weeks in Egypt.

How to Return Home

Now before I finish, I have good news, something that we already know. Now this is the most important part of my book! Because this is about our soul, yours and mine. Our body is temporary, but we keep our soul with us forever. We, our souls, have to go back to where we came from when we die. That's why this part is so important. Do you have anything more important than this?

But we forgot entirely the moment when we were born, when we were pushed out against our will from the most favorable place we ever had, because it was too painful or shocking. This might be the reason why we become mean and angry as we grow older. The moment was shockingly painful or painfully shocking or both that we forgot everything, including this most important one. But clearly it is written in the Bible and in our minds, which means it is written everywhere.

So how do we return home, the home we had to leave against our will and must go back to at all costs called the garden of Eden or simply heaven? Yes, the place where we came from. Yes, this is the most important part of my book.

Actually, we were kicked out of heaven when we were born against our will. That's why we cried so hard. When we die or fade away, we go quietly because we all know that it's no use crying. We tried already and failed. Why bother doing something that didn't and doesn't work?

I have three different ways to achieve this ultimate goal. Why three? Because one is not enough. What if your one and only fails? Again, two are too risky. We need three just in case.

By the way, do you remember a person named Henry Ford? The one who had three generators, in case the first one fails or the second one fails while he's fixing the first. That's why we have to have three keys to solve this important task. I have three keys but can share only the first two. The third one is too personal and private to share with anyone. I do not mind if you have more than three. The more, the better!

Surprisingly, all the secrets of going home are written all over in the Bible, if you look carefully. Also, it is written in our hearts. We carry this with us wherever we go, although the Bible stays at home or in the hotel room.

I do not need to explain the one written in our hearts. Let me explain the one written in the Bible. Then where can we find it? It is written in the early part of Genesis. Just after God gave the absolute authority to govern the garden to the first couple, just like humans are governing and controlling this entire world, we all know what happened after they ate the fruit of the tree of the right and wrong. It is not important who ate first or second. But apparently, the one who was created second ate first according to the Bible. It is not important at all who told them to eat the fruit because only humans are able to talk, besides God, no one else. Have you ever read in the Bible that there are others other than humans that were able to talk?

Maybe they discussed who would eat first. Probably, they were debating who would be the first to disobey the Creator. It was inevitable and destined for humans to eat the fruit when they were given the free will as well as curiosity. But most likely, the brave one ate first. Just guess who? However, it is not important who ate first or second. The fact that both of them ate the fruit itself is important. Then you know the rest of the story.

The real important one comes next. When the angry Creator asked the question to both of them, "Who told you to eat that fruit?" The one who ate first lied to God by pointing her finger at a creature that does not have an ability to talk, and then the one who ate second blamed the one who ate first. Both of them gave exactly the wrong answer to God. But the worst and the most pathetic answer came from the one God created first.

Both of them failed the test, i.e., immediate judgment, miserably and were kicked out of home. The moment when they were kicked out, they lost the power or the ability of eternal youth and started marching toward the aging process, i.e., degenerative changes.

Now that you know the real story, always remember what to say and how to answer at the entrance exam at the gate. First and foremost, do not lie. Be honest. And then do not blame others for your mistake, i.e., your sin. This is the bottom line.

(By the way, if you are an extremely honest person and never lied and never blamed others for your mistakes all of your life and be able to be honest for the rest of your life, having no reason to lie at the Gate, then you have an extremely high probability to enter the Gate.

But even though you are not the kind of person I just described above—meaning you lied and blamed others many times in the past as I did—if you choose to be honest and not blame others from now on for the rest of your life and be honest at the Gate, you still have a very high chance to enter the Gate.

Yes, you lied and blamed others all of your life. But only if you can be honest at the Gate, only God knows what would be the result. Remember, a wise man said long ago, "Never too late." You might be where you want to be all of your life.)

Most likely, we will pass the exam if we know how to give the honest answer alone. We do not have to have the second or the third key, as I recommended. What if the first couple were honest and did not blame the other for their mistakes? I'm sure we might be living in a better condition or better place.

But remember Mr. Henry Ford. You never know. What if we could not erase all those mistakes, i.e., sins, that we made through our entire life just by being honest alone? We need more than one or two. We need to have a backup plan.

Here, the second key is what I call "the back door method," also known as "the doggy hole method." By just looking at the name, many readers already recognized what I'm about to say. If the first one does not work, you look for the back door, waiting for you and me. If the gatekeeper points his finger at other direction, then you will pretend that you are sad and disappointed with some tears in your eyes and turn around and then follow the trail along with the wall. Almost at the opposite side of the front gate, you will find a small hole but big enough for an adult to crawl in. You might have to crawl. That's all you need to do. Trust me, you will find this hole. This is why.

A long, long time ago, before Jesus died, his legal father died first. Then Jesus died, followed by his mother. Quite naturally, they are living happily together now at a place also known as heaven where we all want to join them sooner or later. One day, when his legal father was passing by the front gate, he saw many people failed the test and were turned away. So he went to the opposite side with his shovel. We all know his occupation on earth was a carpenter. He was well trained to dig a hole while he was living in Israel. He made a nice tunnel for us to crawl in. And you know the rest of the story.

One day, the gatekeeper noticed and started seeing many of those who flunked the exam walking around inside the wall with a big smile. The gatekeeper found that the legal father of Jesus made a small hole on the opposite side. The gatekeeper was so furious that he demanded to block the hole and then told him to leave heaven because he disobeyed and violated the rule of God.

The next day, Jesus's legal father was packing his backpack. He told his wife what happened. His wife started packing her backpack. When Jesus heard what was going on, he started packing too. All three MIP (most important people) were leaving the place where they belong. The gatekeeper had to change his mind when he saw all three members of the Holy Family leaving the gate. He had no choice but to ask or beg them not to leave and keep the doggy hole business. He promised not to tell anyone what he knows, including God.

So there is a functioning hole, opposite from the front gate. I have not received any news that the hole closed yet. It is very strange that, once inside, no one came back and told me. So I just assume that it is still functioning.

I have a third key, which I unfortunately cannot share with you because it is too personal and private. So you have to find your own third key or more. I'm sure we, the average and ordinary persons, will successfully enter heaven with a smile.

Finally, as I promised in chapter 1, in my opinion, this is the true meaning of "I am the way, and the truth, and the life, no one comes to the Father but through me" as Jesus taught his disciples in the Gospel of John. If we accept the way it is written, we only see Christians in heaven—no one else other than Christians. How is it possible? No one is allowed to go inside heaven if they are not a Christian. But this is not true. Absolutely not true. This is not what he meant. This is the result that he, the Son of God, did his best to emphasize who he is. He did not mean to discriminate based on religion who goes in or not. Why? Because in heaven, there is no discrimination based on anything, including religion. None whatsoever. We will find the truth the moment when we successfully put the first step into heaven.

We will be surprised and even shocked to find out three things as soon as we step in. First and foremost, you will be shocked to find out where you are. Finally, you are at the place where you want to be all your life. Of course, I'll be shocked too. I'm in heaven. For god's sake, we are in heaven! One, we are shocked. Second, you will be shocked to find the people you thought and believed to be in heaven are not in heaven. You cannot find them in heaven. They are somewhere else, a place called H, not heaven. We are shocked twice. And three, you will be shocked to find out the people you thought should not be in heaven are in heaven. What if you find someone who you thought should be in hell walking around in heaven? You will say, "What the hell is going on here?" Or you will accept what you see, such as people with different religions or people with different sexual orientations. We are shocked thrice.

Heaven does not discriminate your age, your sex, your skin color, your religion, your sexual orientations, your money, etc. As a result, quite so naturally, you will see a lot of people in heaven from different religions or no religion only if you pass the test or the entrance exam or the final judgment, to be exact. Heaven does not discriminate who you are, what you are, or where you are from, as long as you pass the test, the final judgment.

So let's meet one another in heaven with a big smile.

John Chun was born in Korea and raised in the third biggest city called Daegu. Then he came to Michigan about forty years ago and is currently living in Ann Arbor for almost thirty-five years. All his three children graduated from the University of Michigan. So quite naturally, he is a proud and devoted fan of Michigan football and basketball.

John used to play tennis a lot when he was young, but he is spending more time playing golf lately.

As you can tell in the book, John traveled a lot in the past but wants to go back as many times as he can to such places like Rome, Egypt, Spain, and Alaska.

CPSIA information can be obtained
at www.ICGtesting.com
Printed in the USA
BVHW061720310122
627188BV00004BA/15

9 781638 446224